I0414972

No Age Is The New Age:
An Action Plan To AGELESS

A Longevity Guide for Men &Women
25 to 125

Eve Michaels & Karen Norris

Edited by:

Michael Easterling

The information contained in this book is intended to provide helpful and informative material on the subject addressed. It is not intended to serve as a replacement for professional medical advice. Before beginning any diet, exercise, or healthcare program, a healthcare professional should be consulted regarding your specific situation. All nutrient, hormone recommendations and nutritional supplements mentioned in this book are not to be taken without the advice of a medical doctor, naturopathic or anti-aging/integrative medical physician, registered dietitian and/or endocrine specialist.

The content of this book was not endorsed by any individual or corporation. The authors did not receive compensation of any kind for mentioning any products or medical professionals in this book.

© Copyright 2010 by Eve Michaels and Karen Norris

All rights reserved. No part of this publication may be reproduced or transmitted in any form or by any means, electronic or mechanical, including photocopying, recording, or any other information storage and retrieval system without the written permission of the publisher.

This book may be purchased for business or promotional use or for special sales. For information please email: Karen@SimplyAgeless411.com

Printed in the United States of America
by
E &K Publishing, Beverly Hills, California 90212

Library of Congress Cataloging-in-Publication Data

No Age Is The New Age

ISBN - 9781453607787

A New Age Is Here…

INTRODUCTION

(Continued on next page)

(Continued on next page)

(Continued on next page)

INTRODUCTION

Mother Nature designed the human body to live 125 years. It's true. With the inexorable conquest of most cancer and neurological disease on the horizon, many more of us will live to 125 in great health. Imagine being considered middle-aged in your 70s or 80s?

With the advances in modern medicine and the more we learn about our own bodies, living well past what you think is your "prime" is more possible than it's ever been.

In the United States, the current benchmark is 115 years old. Los Angeles resident and super centenarian, Gertrude Baines, was recognized as the oldest person in America. She died from dehydration in 2009 at 115. French woman Jeanne Calment is the longest-living verified human ever recorded. She died in 1997 at age 122. These modern-day Methusalehs always get a mention in the media, with the inevitable question: "What is the secret to your long life?"

With the advances in medicine and nutritional supplements, and a better understanding of how the human body ages and how to reverse or at least slow down that process, the Gertrude Baines and Jeanne Calment's of the world may be too common to warrant such press coverage. Think of it: A century ago there were only a handful of centenarians on earth. Today, there are thought to be 340,000 worldwide. Those numbers are projected to increase to between six and eight million within the next 20-30 years.

Living a long healthy life and perhaps hitting our own centenarian milestones requires a shift in thinking for many of us. Between family and job stress, insomnia, fatigue, smoking, caffeine, environmental effects and the overuse of pharmaceuticals, it's a battle to stay healthy, one that we can lose much too soon if we don't take control of our bodies and send the aging process into retreat.

We've discovered over the years that there is a strong need for an understanding, objective, independent voice that can help consumers decide what the next chapter of their lives will look and feel like. We've done the research. We have the experience. We know what it takes to stay healthy and youthful and we're here to share it. We've already done the heavy lifting and make specific recommendations in this book that will be life changing.

As medical correspondents for our company, www.SimplyAgeless411.com , we recently attended the annual *Physician's Fellowship Medical Conference* hosted by *The American Academy of Anti-Aging,* in Las Vegas, Nevada, where more than 3,000 physicians, many of whom are world renowned, converged for a week to teach and to learn about new medical breakthroughs, technologies and shared experiences. We were there to learn as much as possible to share with our clients and connect with doctors and other experts to whom we could refer our clients.

What we came away with is nothing short of life changing. In *No Age is the New Age,* we will dig deeper into the emerging phenomenon of anti-aging and regenerative medicine, nutrigenomics, vitamins and nutritional supplements, hormonal regeneration, brain rejuvenation, breakthroughs on the horizon and explore the advancements in non-invasive cosmetic rejuvenation.

Certainly, we will grow older, but we can remain in great health with an abundance of strength and vitality. We can age with sharp minds and youthful vigor. And, we can better manage the likelihood of disease. A new age is upon us - it's never too late to start, but it is also never too early.

The latest data suggests that aging begins at twenty-five years old. Making just a few smart changes now can alter the course of your life. As someone who wants to live longer and better, you have to participate in your own anti-aging journey. Low-calorie diets and breaking a sweat at the gym on a regular basis are certainly key elements to a longevity program. But throw in a generous helping of scientific advances, and surpassing Mrs.

Clement's record of 122 starts to look quite possible. One hundred fifty could be within reach.

Like those men and women gathered in Las Vegas at the conference, a growing number of maverick, impeccably-credentialed scientists, physicians, researchers, biogeneticists and nanotechnologists are insisting that the war on aging is a winnable one. They all contend that longer life spans and even biological immortality are scientifically achievable. What's more, it's not a far-off notion of which our great grandchildren will reap the rewards. It's happening, *now,* bubbling just below the surface to potentially help many of us today live much, much longer than we ever thought we could.

"The first person to live to be 150 years old is alive today; indeed, he or she may be about to turn 60," says Aubrey de Grey, the Cambridge University geneticist who has become the spokesman of the anti-aging crusade. "Whether they realize it or not, barring chronic disease, accidents and suicide, most people now 40 years or younger can expect to live at least to 150."

Seems impossible, right? True, some scientists dismiss de Grey's predictions as wildly optimistic, but there are plenty of others who agree with his theories and have joined in the search for what could be a genuine "fountain of youth." Michael Rose, professor of evolutionary biology, is one such disciple.

"I am working on immortality," he says boldly. "Twenty years ago the idea of postponing aging, let alone reversing it, was off-the-wall. Today, there are good reasons for thinking it is fundamentally possible." Rose has made great strides in his research extending the lives of fruit flies; progress in the lab that he's confident will impact the human race just as successfully.

Beyond Rose's lab in Irvine, the most spectacular, encouraging findings are coming out of the genetics labs of large, accredited universities all over the world. Anti-aging researchers are working with living organisms ranging from yeast to worms and mice, in an effort to prove their hypotheses on longevity. Some are breeding their test subjects so their offspring live longer, others are altering genetic makeup to determine what hormones and other supplements can extend life beyond current expectations. Still others have discovered that mice and flies, when put on a near-starvation diet, seem to "switch on" some sort of internal anti-aging mechanism that is connected with Silent Information Regulatory genes, or SIR2.

Just in the past couple of years, researchers at Harvard Medical School and the University of California, Davis, have detected four "cousins" of SIR2 that also seem to play a role in aging and life extension. David Sinclair, director of the Aging Research Lab at Harvard, has called the SIR2 group "as important as any longevity genes discovered so far".

On the food front, some studies have shown that when small mammals are put on ultra-low-calorie diets approaching starvation, they enter states of quasi-suspended animation in which they can move, but apparently cease aging. Even if suspended animation isn't your bag, it's entirely possible that low-calorie foods like kale, blueberries, flax seeds and tofu will help you tack on a few more years.

To get you still closer to your centennial years, it will be essential for laboratories, at both universities and corporations, to discover new, effective treatments for the common ailments of aging, such as cancer, heart disease and diabetes. Recent breakthroughs like "smart drugs" that target tumors or their blood supplies offer some encouragement. As scientists pursue remedies for each specific ailment of aging, right down to wrinkled skin, the efforts may increasingly overlap and shed still more light on the broad process of aging.

Additionally, proponents of extra-long living see a day within the next 10-20 years when stem cell research and nanotechnology really kicks in. In what now seems strictly science fiction, molecular robots could be running through our bodies, continually making repairs and we can be growing our own new body parts when the old ones wear out. Seriously!

Researchers hoping to unlock the secret to ageless living remain very much on the job. And they say they are convinced that the task of keeping the human body going is just as manageable as any other important chore - say, maintaining a home, or a car. Betting that they're wrong could prove perilous. Is their goal really any more implausible than heavier-than-air flight, the nuclear bomb, satellites, computers, space travel and any number of other 20th-century innovations?

Growing older is inevitable, like taxes and the weather. But how you prepare for those years and weather your own aging process is up to you. What we present in this book are all the tools in our arsenal to get you on your own road toward aging beautifully, with vim, vigor and vitality. In short, to being "simply ageless." Looking good and feeling good is not confined to a number. Making just a few smart changes now can alter the course of the rest of your life.

If you are closer to mid-life and beyond, there has never been a better time to reset the dynamics of your thinking and to change the course of your health and emotional well-being. We hope you enjoy this book, learn from it and keep it handy as your journey towards anti-aging begins.

Eve and Karen

PART I:

Hormonal Harmony:

Restoring the Delicate Balance

Chapter One

Ctrl-Alt-Replete:
Time for a Hormonal Reboot?

As a teenager, your voracious appetite, growth spurt, pimples and sudden preoccupation with s-e-x was chalked up to "hormones" by your stressed-out parents, as adolescence set in. Decades later, your mood swings, fatigue, and decreased libido are also the result of hormones, this time rather than raging seem to be going into retirement.

Everything you do - your thoughts, feelings, emotions, physical growth and maintenance is influenced by hormones, throughout your life. Getting to know them and how they work in your body is a good first step toward attacking the aging process. By proactively educating yourself about them, being familiar with signs and symptoms of hormonal imbalance, and finally controlling them is as crucial as anything else you can do for your health and well being. Proper nutrition and exercise are certainly important, but without a healthy balance in hormone levels, none of us can really thrive. Many of the following symptoms could be the result of a hormone imbalance:

- Fatigue, even after an ample amount of sleep

- Depression, for no apparent reason
- Difficulty losing weight
- Inability to concentrate
- Irregular bowel movements
- General lack of stamina
- Loose, saggy skin
- Irritability
- Decreased immunity
- Loss of muscle mass
- Irregular menstrual cycles in women
- Erectile dysfunction in men

Sound familiar? According to Ryan Stanton, MD, a top hormone specialist in Beverly Hills and a medical consultant to SimplyAgeless411, there are several imperative hormones that are affected as you age: **estrogen, progesterone, thyroid hormones, cortisol, testosterone, DHEA, pregnenolone and human growth hormone.**

In the next few chapters of this book, we will introduce you to each of these primary hormones and explain the important roles that they play in your body and the dramatic effects that a decline or imbalance in any one of them can have on your health, your appearance and your personality. Here is a quick rundown of the master hormones that govern our bodies:

Estrogen. The all-important, much-revered (and occasionally maligned) hormone that is many ways ground zero for the healthy, happy woman. It is responsible for those sexy, fertile, strong, peppy, voluptuous characteristics that define women in today's society. However, men need small amounts of estrogen too— without it, they can become sterile and have a low sex drive. Too much estrogen in the male can result in lost muscle tone, a higher voice and diminished energy. **Progesterone** -- primarily a female hormone – should exist in small amounts in men to create just the right balance for youthful, cheerful, calming, steady and well-balanced personality traits.

Thyroid hormones, generated in both sexes, are responsible for regulating all metabolic functions and energy production in the body and brain, such as digestion, healthy liver function and weight control. **Cortisol** gives you energy, helps you handle stress, and enables you to be quick and active. **Testosterone**, the "macho hormone" that men like to brag they have in ample doses, is important to both sexes as it provides muscle tone, strong bones, a healthy libido, mood, and energy. **Human Growth Hormone (HGH)** is a kind of "master switch" hormone that regulates the growth and maintenance of essentially all tissues of the body.

Dehydroepiandrosterone**, or DHEA**, is one of our most powerful hormones made in both men and women. An endogenous steroid – meaning it exists in the body naturally – DHEA is produced by the adrenal glands and also synthesized in the brain. It preserves adrenal function for the immune system and provides numerous anti-aging benefits, such as enhancing muscle mass and skin tone, improving memory, decreasing clinical depression and protecting against certain cancers. **Pregnenolone** is the "memory hormone" that can improve retention, stimulate concentration, clarify thinking and reduce mental fatigue.

Each of us will lose different hormones at different times and rates. Any hormonal imbalance can accelerate the aging process. Who needs that? The good news is that a decline of any hormone is *neither irreparable nor permanent.* In fact, regaining that vital balance is probably easier than you'd think. What it does require is your time and patience to reset the dynamics of your hormonal profile, a "reboot" that can yield amazing results. A successful balance achieved through hormone replacement therapy is like a symphony where each instrument (or hormone) plays a different tune to create a musical masterpiece. It's you, 2.0.

Unfortunately, hormones cannot be replaced through foods or supplements. The only way to safely reset your hormones to younger levels is through hormone supplements, which work to nourish your aging body and brain and stimulate the production of biochemicals such as dopamine, a powerful neurotransmitter that can get you firing on all cylinders again.

From our own experience, and in our discussions with integrative medicine physicians around the world, we have determined that bio-identical hormones are the *best* course of treatment in hormone replacement. Bio-identical hormones are plant-based hormone supplements that have the same molecular structure as those that occur naturally in the body. They are far safer than traditional hormone therapies, which are often synthetically produced.

Many pharmaceutical companies are now creating new bio-identical hormone products; however, they are generally a "one size fits all" approach containing "standard doses" that assume our bodies are all the same, which of course, isn't the case. A "standard dose" can be too much for one person and not enough for another. Any customized system of hormone replacement is the best way to ensure you get the standard dose your body needs.

You should begin by making an appointment for a hormonal profile. The test you schedule will allow you to see exactly which hormones are not functioning properly. At that time the doctor will write you a prescription for the exact amount of bio-identical hormones that your body needs to achieve a healthy balance.

More often than not, you will have your prescriptions filled at a compounding pharmacy, which is usually a separate division of your regular pharmacy that specializes in customized solutions per a physician's directive. Believe it or not, the cost to have your own prescription made up by a compounding pharmacy is about the same as the pre-packaged pharmaceutical one-size-fits-all brands that you get at the regular pharmacy counter. And like the ready-made kind, those that are compounded just for your body are also available in different forms, the most popular being creams, gels, skin patches, under-the-tongue drops, vaginal suppositories and capsules.

Finding Dr. Right

Despite the changing attitudes, many primary care physicians are not familiar with bio-identical hormone replacement, and how natural hormones can help many problems associated with the aging process in both men and women. It wasn't part of their academic curricula, and is still resisted as a course of treatment by some simply because it falls outside the boundaries of what they consider to be traditional medicine. There are numerous, qualified specialists listed on our website, *www.SimplyAgeless411.com*. The information is yours for the taking. You may also seek a referral from your internist or gynecologist. They may refer you to an endocrinologist because they officially specialize in hormones, but be aware that many of them specialize in diabetes and have not had extensive experience treating and working with natural bio-identical hormone replacement. They may recommend synthetic hormones developed by pharmaceutical companies, *which is not what you want to do.*

One of the reasons that we developed our website *www.SimplyAgeless411.com* is to give you free access to doctors who specialize in the field of anti-aging/integrative medicine. We do not receive any kind of fees or compensation from any of the medical professionals listed on our site. Our goal is simply to help people get to the right doctors.

In any case, you want to make sure your doctor has plenty of clinical experience with all hormone deficiencies and multiple-hormone treatments. A highly skilled and experienced anti-aging physician develops a kind of sixth sense that allows them to have a good idea what to investigate more closely about you as soon as you walk into the room.

Your face, hands, skin, hair, eyes, feet, the silhouette of your body, your energy level, the way you walk, the pitch, tone and levity of your voice, the clarity of your thinking, your overall demeanor and look—all of these are tell-tale signs of one or more hormone deficiencies. That initial consult will help the doctor form a preliminary diagnosis, which can be confirmed after the hormonal profile, which typically consists of testing of the blood, urine and oftentimes, saliva.

Remember, no matter how many specialists you consult, you will always be the best expert on your own body. Once you understand how to tune in and really listen to what your body is telling you, it is amazing how easy it can be to identify what it needs. It also creates a more robust dialogue with your doctor that enhances their ability to treat you.

Chapter Two

The Masters:
Our Most Valuable Hormones

The Thyroid Rules

It is estimated that between 30 percent to as much as 80 percent of the world's population (both men and women) has some degree of low thyroid function (Hypothyroidism). Even more unfortunate is the fact that this imbalance -- which affects so many aspects of health -- is frequently either misdiagnosed, misunderstood, or completely overlooked. Hypothyroidism can occur for a host of reasons. It can be congenital, can present at menopause or just after, or be the result of exposure to certain viruses, an iodine deficiency, a direct physical trauma to the thyroid gland itself, a head trauma effecting the pituitary, autoimmune disease, or environmental toxins.

Common symptoms of Hypothyroidism include:
- Fatigue
- Accelerated aging
- Weight gain
- Cold dry skin

- Joint and muscle pain (even Fibromyalgia)
- Constipation
- Memory loss
- Brain fog, inability to concentrate
- Hair thinning/loss

Since many doctors misdiagnose hypothyroidism, we asked a well-known hormone specialist for the breakdown of tests that should be performed for a comprehensive thyroid evaluation.

Your initial lab tests (blood work) should include:

Thyroid stimulating hormone (TSH), free thyroxine (T4), free tri-iodothyronine (T3), and reverse tri-iodothyronine (rT3) levels. TSH is produced by the pituitary gland and stimulates the thyroid gland to produce T4 and T3, the active thyroid hormones. Insufficient production of any one of these can lead to hypothyroidism. On the other hand, reverse T3 is an *inactive* form of T3 and overproduction of this form of thyroid hormone can also cause hypothyroidism.

Treatment for Hypothyroidism includes:

Simply replacing with Bio-identical T4, which is available in pill form. Because many people seem to have a more difficult time converting T4 to T3 -- which is actually the more active form -- T3 replacement is often recommended as well. Armour Thyroid is a

Bio-identical thyroid replacement medication that is commonly prescribed by specialists because it contains both T4 and T3. This treatment is usually very effective and the results can be quick and dramatic.

We can tell you firsthand that when the thyroid is working correctly it energizes the cells and organs by stimulating the mitochondria in the body – the "power plants" that fuel cellular rejuvenation. Thyroid hormones warm the body, especially the extremities, and prevent sensitivity to hot and cold. They stave off morning fatigue. Thyroid hormones also stabilize mental alertness and acuity and protect the kidneys, the digestive and immune systems, the heart, arteries and virtually all tissues that compromise the innermost workings of the human body. In short, the thyroid is a major player in your hormone health.

Cortisol and the Adrenal Glands

Cortisol is produced by the adrenal glands which sit on top of the kidneys. Cortisol is considered the main "stress" hormone and helps us manage both physical and psychological pressures. When cortisol levels rise in response to stressors, we get a boost of energy, our memory is sharper, and we are more motivated - all positive outcomes. It boosts dopamine-related chemicals, giving us more juice when are brains seem to be running low on fuel.

Constant stress, however, can cause an overproduction of cortisol, which can have adverse and even toxic effects, including the destruction of brain cells. Here are signs of too much Cortisol:

Common signs & symptoms of elevated cortisol levels:
- Depression
- Memory malfunction
- Anxiety
- Fatigue
- Stomach ulcers
- High blood pressure
- Elevated cholesterol
- Weight gain
- Food & alcohol cravings
- Insulin resistance
- Heart disease
- Osteoporosis
- Frequent illnesses

The first step in reducing high levels of cortisol is through proper nutrition and exercise and adequate sleep. Cut back on salt, simple sugars and white flour products, eat more frequent smaller meals (at least four a day), curb your alcohol intake, and exercise at least three times a week for at least 20-30 minutes, depending on intensity.

When life throws you too many curves, as it will do on occasion, and you can't seem to escape stress and anxiety or manage it through diet and exercise, the adrenal glands eventually become worn out. Cortisol levels drop below the threshold necessary to handle stress and the result is what is medically referred to as "Adrenal Fatigue."

Here are symptoms of low Cortisol or Adrenal Fatigue:

- Stress intolerance
- Chronic Fatigue Syndrome
- Intolerance to cold temperatures
- Onset of new allergies
- Loss of stamina
- Weight gain (from poor blood sugar regulation)
- Aches and pains, including Fibromyalgia
- Prolonged illnesses and common colds
- Alcoholism
- Depression
- Rheumatoid arthritis
- Heart disease
- Insomnia
- Asthma

Again, because cortisol affects other hormones, when it is too low it can cause hypothyroidism because it is necessary for the production and function of thyroid hormones.

According to Beverly Hills hormone specialist, Ryan Stanton, MD, the best treatment for low cortisol levels is a standard lab test followed by bio-identical replacement therapy.

Although blood, urine, and saliva tests exist, blood testing is still the gold standard when diagnosing and treating most illnesses in the body, including hormone depletion. Because cortisol levels are highest in the morning (about an hour after awakening) and then drop sharply for about the next 4-5 hours, then very slowly drop throughout the rest of the day, it is recommended to draw blood both first thing in the morning, and again late in the afternoon. Adrenal corticotrophin hormone (ACTH) is produced by the pituitary and stimulates the adrenals to produce cortisol. Testing ACTH levels in the blood will also help your physician determine if the hormone depletion resides in the pituitary or the adrenal glands.

As with thyroid deficiencies we discussed earlier, treatment for adrenal fatigue is as simple as bioidentically replacing the cortisol hormone with a pill produced by your compounding pharmacy expressly for your body. Not only does this replenish the body with the needed hormone, but it also gives the adrenals a chance to recover and relax after working overtime. As always, exercise and eating right are timeworn methods of stress relief.

Estrogen – Getting Your Sexy Back

In many ways, estrogen is the biological essence of a woman. It creates the female shape (breasts, hips, pelvis and even face) and controls the menstrual cycle. It keeps skin smooth and unwrinkled, prevents excess hair growth and keeps the vagina lubricated. It enhances sexual desire, increases physical endurance and contributes to a positive mood. Estrogen keeps the eyes and mouth moist and the eyes shining bright.

It produces a positive mood—happiness, enthusiasm, and zeal—and can prevent chemical depression. Estrogen develops sexual desire and the desire to love. It fights fatigue, reduces the risk of heart disease, retards osteoporosis, protects the brain by keeping the neurons firing, keeps the joints healthy and supports immune function.

At puberty, a woman's ovaries start producing significant amounts of estrogen; however, as a woman's hormone levels begin to decline -- which can occur as early as the late 20s -- the ovaries dramatically decrease production. Fat tissue becomes the predominant source of estrogen. A woman without sufficient estrogen may experience hair loss, fine wrinkles around the eyes and mouth, especially above the lips and experience dry, irritated eyes.

Other dramatic symptoms can include insomnia, sagging breasts and loss of the overall plumpness that adds the curves to your figure at the chest, hips and pelvis. Women may also experience a lack of sexual desire and vaginal dryness, which can result in painful intercourse without external lubrication. A deficiency of estrogen can cause lethargy, depression, and a host of menstrual problems, such as severe cramping and irregular cycles that are either too short or too long.

Lowered estrogen levels are the source of many of the familiar symptoms of menopause, most frequently the infamous "hot flashes". Younger women might also get hot flashes during menstruation if their estrogen levels are too low. There are, in fact, more than 400 tissue systems throughout the body where estrogen has a major impact. We recommend that women begin monitoring their estrogen levels in their late 20s to get a baseline reading.

Your body makes three main estrogens:
- E1 - called Estrone. Many doctors believe it may be related to an increase in breast and uterine cancer.

- E2 – called Estradiol. It helps maintain your memory, bone health and aids in the protection from heart disease.

- E3 – called Estriol. Considerable evidence exists to show that it may protect against breast cancer.

Have your physician measure all three types of estrogen in your blood profile. "It is important for optimal health that your hormone replacement therapy be comprised of estradiol and estriol (bi-est) and *not* contain estrone," says world-renowned leading integrative medical physician and hormone and breast cancer specialist, Pamela Smith, MD.

Bioidentical estrogen comes in several types of delivery systems: cream or gel applied to the skin, patches, sublingual drops, vaginal suppositories and oral capsules (oral capsules are not recommended by most physicians because of poor absorption rates.) At the time of the writing of this book, the delivery systems of choice recommended by most physicians are the gels and creams; however, new technologies are being developed every day. Ask your physician about the latest advancements in estrogen delivery systems, and which one is right for you.

To the men out there, take note: estrogen also plays a very important role in your hormonal profile. It is important to have the correct ratio of estrogen to testosterone. Low estrogen can cause infertility and too much can increase the risk of a heart attack or stroke. A knowledgeable doctor will know to check both the estrogen and testosterone levels in a man's hormonal profile.

Overall, for both men and women, your physician will do a hormonal profile on your blood tests to determine your estrogen levels and recommend bio-identical hormone supplementation to regulate them if the levels are too high or too low.

Can Soy Milk & Tofu Increase Estrogen Levels Naturally?

In a word, "No." Soy is a wonderful plant. We eat and enjoy many soy products such as tofu, tempeh, miso and soymilk. These products contain natural hormone-like compounds readily absorbed into the body. These compounds known as phyto-estrogens or isoflavones, go by the name of genistein, daidzein and glycitein. According to a top hormone specialist Uzzi Reiss, MD, these isoflavones are "weak chemicals."

"They are a thousand times weaker than the hormones in our bodies, Dr. Reiss explains. "When you eat soy, you assimilate these compounds. They get into your bloodstream and may generate some benefits. These benefits, however, are not nearly as significant as those that result from taking bio-identical hormones."

Progesterone – The Hormonal Harmonizer

Progesterone is made primarily in the ovaries during pregnancy. The adrenal glands also produce small quantities of the hormone in both men and women. Additionally in men, the testicles produce a small amount. Progesterone protects the heart and bones and has anti-cancer properties, particularly against endometrial and breast cancer. It relaxes, calms, reduces worry and nervousness and provides better and deeper sleep. It can trigger a sense of deep tranquility and inner peace. Who doesn't want that?

Progesterone provides many major protective functions to the body, and perhaps most important, it balances estrogen levels in both men and women. Anytime that the estrogen level rises in the body you want to have progesterone there to offset it. In women, progesterone affects many tissues other than the uterus including the urinary tract, heart, blood vessels, breasts, bones, hair, skin, pelvic muscles, and brain.

Progesterone is produced primarily after ovulation by the empty egg sac. Logically, if a woman doesn't ovulate, her body creates much less progesterone. There are several other (less common) explanations for low or declining progesterone levels, including high cortisol levels, certain synthetic chemicals that incompletely mimic and interfere with estrogen and luteal phase defects, where you ovulate but still don't produce an adequate amount of progesterone. All these scenarios lead to an imbalance between estrogen and progesterone. As mentioned previously, all hormones -- especially estrogens and progesterone in this regard -- should be kept in a very harmonious, tight critical balance for us to function and feel our best.

Signs and Symptoms of Low Progesterone in women:
- Uterine fibroids
- Fibrocystic breasts
- Insomnia
- Weight gain
- Anxiety
- Fatigue
- Excessive menstrual bleeding
- Increased risk of breast cancer

Signs and Symptoms of Low Progesterone in men:
- Increased body fat
- Decreased libido
- Enlarged prostate

Your physician will do a hormonal profile on your blood tests to determine your progesterone levels, and will recommend bio-identical hormone supplementation if your levels are too high or low. "For women, your initial tests should include an Ovulation Self Test, which can be purchased at any pharmacy and used at home, before you have the blood test at your doctor's office," Dr. Stanton recommends. "Any woman in her mid-30s or above should use this test to check whether she is ovulating or not, and if so, if it is regular.

This will give the first clue to dropping progesterone levels. Blood tests should look at progesterone and estradiol levels when they are peaked, around day 21 of your menstrual cycle, follicle stimulating hormone (FSH), which is the hormone produced by the pituitary that stimulates the ovaries to produce more estrogen, should also be checked around day 21, testosterone and thyroid hormone levels, and finally cortisol levels in the early morning and late afternoon." For men, progesterone levels are tested in the standard hormonal profile evaluation.

Dr. Stanton recommends using bio-identical progesterone replacement therapy as a treatment for low levels of the hormone. "Usually a cream applied once a day can rebalance progesterone with estrogen," he says. "I recommend creams over pills because when taken orally, the medication is absorbed by the stomach and passes through the liver where sometimes as much as 90 percent of the medication is metabolized to an inactive form. This can be especially hard on the liver and could eventually lead to liver disease." Dr. Stanton says that topicals can be found at any standard or compounding pharmacy.

"T" For Two: Testosterone is Important to Both Men AND Women

If estrogen is the biological essence of a woman, testosterone has been called a man's "hormone of virility." While this is true, it is important to realize its importance to both men *and* women. Testosterone stimulates the libido in both sexes. For men, testosterone is necessary for erections, ejaculations and fertility, and plays a significant role as men get older with dealing with male menopause (more on that later). In both sexes, testosterone stimulates the feeling of love and sexuality.

In both sexes, testosterone protects the heart and arteries and reduces the risk of heart disease. It can also counter high cholesterol and angina. It also protects the pancreas, kidneys and digestive organs. It prevents joint and muscle pain, osteoporosis and, in men, obesity. Listen up guys—it can also stop those outbursts of excessive sweat that correspond to hot flashes in women. It builds muscle and increases muscle tone, preserves bone mass and reduces fat, including cellulite, firming up the body's contours.

It tightens and tones the skin, preventing dryness and small wrinkles. In both sexes, testosterone increases your ability to withstand stress and reduces anxiety, depression, and excessive emotional outbursts. It provides energy and endurance and contributes to an overall good mood. It helps you take initiative and employ leadership qualities and makes you assertive, audacious and mentally tenacious. It helps you face difficulties and helps put petty annoyances of everyday life into perspective.

Symptoms of Low Testosterone

Without enough testosterone you may suffer a loss of sexual desire. Men have a tendency to have weaker erections and ejaculations, and women will lose clitoral sensitivity. Men's penises can also get flabby and they may notice a reduction in the size of their testicles, which is quite a traumatic experience for them, especially if they don't know what's happening, and why.

In both sexes, when testosterone levels are low, a feeling of fatigue and malaise may occur, day and night. A loss of self-confidence and a tendency toward depression, anxiety and emotional outbursts may result. Sleep might be agitated and restless, memory and creativity is compromised, and thinking and attitudes borders on the rigid. Some may also notice flabby cheek muscles, a pallor to the skin, dry eyes, and tiny wrinkles on the cheeks and eyes. A lack of testosterone precipitates a "soft" appearance, with a hunched back, loose stomach and flabby hips. Men will notice thin and poorly developed mustaches and beards and a loss of hair on the torso.

Not so Macho: Too Much Testosterone Can Also Be a Problem

World renowned celebrity golf pro, Tiger Woods, was in the news in 2010 with reports of erratic behavior with women and a reported sexual addiction. It's too easy to dismiss the behavior as the loutish scheming of a wealthy, overindulged star athlete on a power trip. We at *SimplyAgeless411,* along with many medical professionals, believe that a pathological cause and effect existed that shaped the golfers thinking and action. Genetics, and a potential hormonal imbalance -- specifically, naturally high testosterone levels -- contributed to his misguided moral compass.

Genetics certainly plays some role in determining how much testosterone men produce, but according to *New Scientist* magazine, culture, fatherhood and other factors can "tinker" with levels over a lifetime and "disrupt family life." The *New Scientist* article goes on to say that evidence is 'piling up" that naturally high testosterone levels affects mating and parenting in humans and that the father of young children is a good candidate to seek treatment to lower levels of the testosterone hormone.

"Not only are you less likely to forget the child and pursue some other mating opportunity, but your temper may be lowered," says Harvard University anthropologist Peter Ellison. Other signs of naturally high testosterone levels in both women include aggressive and "pushy" behavior, a hyper-critical attitude toward family, friends and employees, a perfectionistic bent, a highly agitated state of mind, excessively oily skin on face and back, hair growing in unusual places, loss of hair on the head and an increase in facial hair.

The best way to confirm testosterone imbalances is to have your physician measure your blood for three levels testosterone: *Total testosterone, Free testosterone* and *BioAvailable* testosterone. *Total testosterone* is the total amount in the blood, but the portion bound to the protein called "sex hormone" binding globulin cannot be used by the cells. *Free testosterone* is the amount floating free that the cells can access, which makes it a better measure of useful testosterone, but it does not consider the usable portion loosely bound to albumin. *Bioavailable* is the amount floating free compounded with the amount that is loosely bound to albumin that can be used by the cells. This is perhaps the most useful number.

Again, across the board, the treatment of choice for testosterone deficiencies among integrative medical doctors is bio-identical hormone therapy. As with other bio-identical hormones, testosterone therapy is available in prescriptive-grade patches, gels, creams, pills, pellets and injections. *Do not even consider* dosing yourself with over-the-counter supplements. The results could be life-threatening and do far more damage than good.

DHEA: First Chair in the Hormonal Orchestra

DHEA is one of the body's most abundant hormones. In both men and women DHEA works to help your body repair itself and promote improved immune system functions and anti-aging effects, as well as enhanced energy and weight control. DHEA is naturally produced in the brain and the adrenal glands, and provides significant benefits to address a wide array of health concerns. DHEA can increase testosterone levels, increase muscle mass, improve memory, decrease body fat, decrease depression, lower cholesterol levels and insulin levels and protect against breast cancer. Over a lifetime, your body will secrete more DHEA than any other hormone. In young adults, its concentration in the blood is almost 20 times higher than any other hormone. DHEA's unique ability to convert into other hormones when necessary is its main job, a most important one.

DHEA does the following:

- Increases human growth hormone (HGH)
- Increases allopregnenolone and endorphins; this explains why supplementing DHEA makes us feel calm.
- Converts into estrogen when needed
- Converts into other androgens, like testosterone, but only in specific cells designed for this conversion
- Increases progesterone levels when needed
- Supports the adrenal glands by reducing cortisol and thereby reducing stress
- Can correct defects associated with thyroid diseases such as Graves' disease and Hashimoto's disease
- Improves fertility treatment response in women

Your body's production of DHEA reaches its peak between the ages of 20 and 30, and then begins a slow decent. By the age of 60, production of DHEA is only at 5 percent of its peak. As we mentioned earlier, all hormones are interdependent, which is why understanding and embracing the full scope of hormone replacement needs to be understood. Replacing DHEA without replacing other hormones is ineffective: remember it is just one instrument in the orchestra.

Have your integrative medical physician measure your DHEA levels through a blood or saliva test to determine if supplementation is needed. Unlike the other master hormones, DHEA can be purchased in medical grade from your physician or at a reputable health food store. We like to recommend 7-Keto DHEA because it is a form of DHEA that does not convert into testosterone which, in some people has been shown to cause side effects such as acne and anxiety.

HGH – Human Growth Hormone – Reversing the Aging Process

Human Growth Hormone (HGH) is one of the biggest breakthroughs in anti-aging medicine and may well be the medical community's proverbial fountain of youth. Thousands of studies confirm that raising HGH levels can help prevent and even *reverse* the aging process. Raising HGH levels has also been known to turn around diminished mental capacity and cognition, as well as create sharper vision and improved sleep.

Perhaps a more accurate term for HGH would be "healing" or "anti-aging" hormone. Growth hormone is naturally produced by our pituitary gland and is essential for bone and organ growth in our youth. Although HGH is no longer needed for growth after reaching adulthood, HGH is essential for many other vital functions, and the significantly lowered levels seen as we age are correlated with everything from depleted energy, cardiovascular disease, weight gain (fat), decreased muscle mass, wrinkles, and most other conditions associated with aging. According to a recent report from Kent Holtorf, MD, CEO of The Hormone & Longevity Center in Torrance, California, Human Growth hormone diminishes rapidly after the age of 30, and it is this rapid decline that results in many negative aspects of aging, including increased body fat, decreased muscle mass, increased wrinkles, cancer, and heart disease.

"It is found that growth hormone deficient patients have almost 50 percent higher rate of death from heart disease than those with more optimal levels," Dr. Holtorf explains. "In a 1990 *New England Journal of Medicine* article, Daniel Rudman, MD, reported on his study with the use of human growth hormone in elderly veterans. He discovered that their body fat and wrinkles decreased and lean muscle mass, strength, and bone density increased. The usual progression of aging was halted and reversed by bringing an individual's growth hormone to a more optimal (youthful) level."

Dr. Rudman's findings are excerpted here:

"The effects of six months of human growth hormone on lean body mass and adipose tissue reversed the equivalent of changes

incurred during 10-20 years of aging. The overall deterioration of the body that comes with growing old is not inevitable...We now realize that some aspects of it can be prevented or reversed."
- Dr. Daniel Rudman, MD - New England Journal of Medicine

Dr. Holtorf cites another landmark study from 1999 conducted by the National Institute on Aging to refute or substantiate Dr. Rudman's findings, and to extend his study by measuring other parameters. This study was a double-blind, placebo-controlled, multi-center trial in both men and women with a large number of patients, and involved not only growth hormone but also estrogen, progesterone and testosterone. The results not only confirmed the benefits of growth hormone, but also demonstrated that introducing estrogen/progesterone and testosterone improved its efficacy. After two months, patients participating in the study were observed and presented the following dramatic effects:

<u>Physical Signs</u>
- Less wrinkles on face (75.5%)
- Less sagging skin on face and neck (67%)
- Firmer muscles (60.7%)
- Less body fat (48%)
- Better skin (thicker) (34.5%)
- Thicker head hair (28.1%)

Emotional/mental

- Improved emotional state (71.4%)
- Increased energy (86.8%)
- Improved physical stamina (86.04%)
- Increased ability to stay up late (82.5%)
- Improved resistance to stress ((83.7%)
- Significantly decreased Anxiety (calmer) (73.5%)
- Improved assertiveness (73.1%)
- Improved sense of power (77.8%)
- Improved self-esteem (50%)
- Depression improved or eliminated (82.7%)
- Improved sociability (77.8%)
- Decreased tendency to give sharp verbal retorts (71.0%)

This study and numerous others demonstrate that treatment with growth hormone results in significant improvements in both physical appearance and in emotional and mental well-being, Dr. Holtorf says. "The enhancement in quality-of-life with the use of Growth Hormone is truly remarkable."

Signs and Symptoms of Low HGH:

- Fatigue
- Low libido
- Weight gain (especially abdominal fat)
- Dry & thinning skin

- Decreased stamina &/or strength
- Depressed immune system & frequent colds
- Osteoporosis
- Joint & muscle aches and pains
- Slowed thinking/mentation
- Increased risk of Heart disease
- Increased risk of Strokes

According to top hormone specialist, Ryan Stanton, MD, HGH can be evaluated through a routine blood test measuring levels of Insulin-like Growth Factor 1 (IGF-1), a protein that is produced in response to stimulation by HGH. IGF-1 provides a better overall picture of HGH levels on average rather than just the HGH levels itself at the time of the test, which fluctuates widely on any given time of day. Dr. Stanton cautions that patients who have the test may still be considered having low levels even if within the labs "normal range." "It could be if the patient is experiencing some of the symptoms and/or the occupation and lifestyle of the patent simply require a higher level to maintain," Dr. Stanton explains.

Treatment for low HGH includes: Prescribing bio-identical human growth hormone replacement therapy, only effective as a daily subcutaneous injection (similar to insulin) given anywhere between 3 to 6 days per week. Be aware that there are many ineffective "phony" products on the market (especially through the internet) that make claims of having HGH properties, and are available in either pill or liquid spray form. Dr. Stanton warns that these products may not be safe or produce satisfactory results. It is always best to consult your doctor when beginning any hormone therapy treatment.

Anti-aging physicians usually try to supplement HGH to boost your IGF-1 levels to the upper 25 percent of the normal range, achieving effects while still keeping the levels within the physiologic normal range. This practice also greatly minimizes the most common potential side effects, such as water retention and aching joints. Finally, despite a lot of discussion and concern that HGH supplementation may cause cancer, there is *not a single case reported or study that concluded this to be true*!

It always amazed us when we read news reports or watch an expose on *60 minutes* warning of the dangers and increased cancer risks associated with HGH. The reality is that there has *never been one case of cancer* or any other disease directly linked to the physician-monitored use of HGH. Another vast misconception about HGH is that it is cost prohibitive for the average patient. Virtually everyone we have spoken to about HGH is convinced that the average cost of HGH is approximately $1,000 per vial. For the record, the average cost of one 5.8 mg. bottle of HGH, (using Omnitrope, which is a standard brand) has an average cost in the U.S. of approximately $300-$400 per bottle if purchased through your physician. If a small amount is used once a day, this will last the average person about a month. Once again, *do not use HGH without consulting with your physician.*

You Must Remember This: Pregnenolone

If you were to build a brain from scratch, the key ingredient would be pregnenolone. This hormone aids in the building, performance and maintenance of the brain. Produced in the adrenal glands and the brain itself, pregnenolone is a precursor of all of the adrenal and sex hormones. It is the most abundant hormone in the brain. Pregnenolone's concentration in the brain is seventy-five times higher than in the blood. Because pregnenolone feeds production of so many other hormones, an insufficient level creates a domino effect and compromises the levels of other hormones in the body.

Alertness – One of the ways that antidepressant medications like Prozac work is by increasing the level of pregnenolone in the brain. Drinking alcohol increases the level of pregnenolone in the brain. This may not mean anything to you at first, but it shows just how brilliant the brain is. Alcohol acts as a sedative when consumed. As a result, your brain increases production of pregnenolone to decrease the sedative effect.

Your body also increases pregnenolone levels when you take medications such as Valium, to counteract the sedation. What this all means is, whatever sedation and alcohol take away from you, pregnenolone hands back. It literally protects the brain from being over sedated. Because it reduces fear and promotes social confidence, pregnenolone is often present in high amounts in gregarious, outgoing individuals, and a deficit in those with social phobias.

Dr. Reiss accounts in his latest book, The *Natural SuperWoman* about his favorite dog, 17-year old chow. Five years ago the beloved pet began suffering from arthritis, which slowed her down substantially. Dr. Reiss began administering some of the hormone replacement technology he provides for his patients, and was delighted to see its effects. "By giving her 25 milligrams of DHEA each day, and then upping the dosage to 50 milligrams, then 100, and finally 200 after several weeks, she was more alert, sociable and interested in her surroundings, and even began tracking birds she saw on television!" The arthritis also improved and she was able to go on long walks with her owner, something she hadn't been able to do in years. She simply responded favorably to changes in her hormonal profile.

We share this story not to begin a trend of treating dogs with bio-identical hormones, but because it colors the discussion of the potential efficacy of DHEA and pregnenolone in humans.

Your physician can measure your pregnenolone levels when you have your hormone profile tested. The same blood test run for other hormone levels can yield results for pregnenolone. If you are advised to begin taking a supplement, medical grade pregnenolone is available from your physician or at a reputable health food store. The standard beginning does is a 50 mg tablet every day.

To verify our findings and dig a little deeper, we took some time to pick the brain of one of the premiere experts on anti-aging and the role hormones play. Wayne Wightman, MD is one of the top anti-aging physicians and hormone specialists in the country. His office is located in the Los Angeles suburb of Torrance, California. He is also our own personal physician who has brought us both back from the brink of hormonal madness and continues to introduce us to the latest advancements in the world of anti-aging and regenerative medicine.

He is a physician partner at the Holtorf Medical Group, which is owned by Dr. Holtorf. Dr. Wightman is a former emergency room medical doctor and pharmacist. If you have to fly around the world (and many people do) to get an appointment with one of these doctors, it is worth the trip to become hormonally and nutritionally balanced for the rest of your life.

SimplyAgeless411:   Thank you so much for meeting with us today, Dr. Wightman. Can you give us a bit of insight about any new treatments and therapies on the horizon in the world of anti-aging and regenerative medicine?

Dr. WW: One new treatment that we are having a lot of success with is IV Vitamin Therapy (or intravenous vitamin therapy). This is a means by which a healthy and safe dose of nutrients are given to a patient through their circulatory system through an IV. Vitamins, minerals, and amino acids are put directly into the bloodstream, which guarantees maximum absorption.

When vitamins are taken by mouth, digestion may not extract the optimal amount of the nutrients. Also, some people don't like to take pills, so they come in once a week for treatment and leave feeling fantastic. We're seeing real benefits with this delivery method of vitamins and nutritional supplements such as glutathione, Vitamin C along other nutrients for things like memory and sex drive and improving sports performance. People who travel to other countries and spend many hours on a plane find that IV vitamin therapy strengthens their immune system so that they do not get sick when they travel.

SimplyAgeless411: How long does it take and how much does it cost?

Dr. WW. It takes about an hour for the IV therapy session and the results last for about a week. The cost is roughly $150 per session.

SimplyAgeless411: Is the IV treatment used for anything other than vitamins?

Dr. WW: Yes, we are using it for the treatment of pain management, detoxification, removal of lead and heavy metals, strengthening the immune system and chronic fatigue syndrome.

SimplyAgeless411: You've been treating patients for many years, can you tell us about one of these hormone treatments that have a significant impact on the way we age?

Dr. WW: Well, there are several that top the list such as the treatment for the thyroid, however, the one that comes to mind that has a tremendous impact on how we age is Growth Hormone. It truly is, in my opinion, "The Ultimate Repair Hormone." There have been numerous studies that confirm that raising GH levels can help prevent and even reverse the aging process. Raising GH levels has been known to reverse a decline in memory and cognitive performance, as well as create sharper vision and improved sleep. It also improves the texture of the skin, improves muscle tone, boosts immunity and increases energy and a positive overall sense of well-being.

GH also improves bone density and has a positive effect on the aesthetic bone structure of the face. Facial bone structure changes dramatically with age resulting in sagging skin. Taking GH can help preserve your organic facial structure. GH is just an amazing hormone and our patients love the results it provides. We only recommend it to our patients who are actually low in this hormone and need to bring their levels back to a normal state.

SimplyAgeless411: I know there are pills and all kinds of methods that people use to take growth hormone, however, the only method that works is via an injection that people can administer to themselves at home with a prescription from their doctor, is this correct?

Dr. WW: Yes, that is correct. No other form of growth hormone will work effectively.

SimplyAgeless411: Many people think that obtaining the vials and needles from the doctor's office is very expensive…say over a thousand dollars a bottle. Is this true?

Dr. WW: The average cost of a vial of Growth Hormone in this area is about $380 for a vial that lasts about a month. The small needles are priced around $50, which is enough to last for about a month.

SimplyAgeless411: Dr. Wightman, new advancements in medical research are happening so quickly, especially in the area of nanotechnology and stem cell research, in this new world of medicine, what is the life span now of the average middle aged person?

Dr. WW: Well, the human body was designed to live to the age of 120. With medical research advancing so quickly and with many people finally embracing the world of anti-aging and regenerative medicine, in the next few years we will see a lot more people living in great health to the age of 120 and beyond.

SimplyAgeless411: Wow! These are fascinating times that we live in and it is so exciting that we will all be experiencing this anti-aging journey together. Thank you so much for your time today, Dr. Wightman.

Chapter Three

Beating the Pauses:

Male Menopause & Female

Menopause - What You Need To

Know...

Female Menopause – The Ultimate Age Accelerator That You Can Stop Now

The days of women going into a rapid freefall of aging and deterioration beginning at thirty-five are over. At least they can be... if you're a flexible thinker. We are here to let you know that a new age is here. Forget everything you thought you knew about women and menopause. Around the world physicians are discovering new breakthroughs every day, and are creating new modalities to keep our hormones at optimal levels throughout our lifetime. Ladies, your attention, please.

Doctors have discovered that menopause is not associated with any particular age: It simply marks the decline in the production of some of our primary hormones such as progesterone, estrogen, thyroid, DHEA, Cortisol, HGH and pregnenolone (all covered in detail in Chapter 2). Many women think that menopause starts around middle age, however, when you begin to experience symptoms, your pause is already in the middle of its course. According to many hormone specialists that we have interviewed, menopause actually begins in your early to mid-thirties (peri-menopause) and can take as many as 10 to 15 years to fully bloom.

The bottom line is this: Women in their thirties are already going into partial menopause and without early intervention; a loss of progesterone can cause agitation, moodiness and increase the effects of PMS. By the time you reach 50, you will most likely feel some of these symptoms of the loss of estrogen, which include:

- Fatigue & weight gain
- Attention deficiencies
- Vaginal dryness
- Failure to ovulate
- Hair loss
- Hot flashes
- Loss of skin tone and elasticity
- Rapidly aged appearance
- Bone weakness
- Loss of libido

The decline in hormones cause a cascade of symptoms, leaving women feeling both hungry and tired: They eat more junk food to stay alert and exercise less due to fatigue. Sounds pretty scary, right? Can you just imagine how women have survived this all these years? Those days are over! It is now possible to stay happy, healthy, youthful, and energetic throughout an entire lifetime.

Imagine a new generation of 40 and 50 somethings who stay beautiful, continue to inspire others and contribute to society until, let's say…100? Yes…it's possible. It may take some time for people to embrace new technologies, and sadly, many people never will, nonetheless, a new day is dawning and those who jump on board will reap the rewards beyond measure.

The first step is to find a good doctor who will be your partner. Try to choose one with a specialty in bio-identical hormone replacement. We've spent months scouring the country to provide the names and contact information of these physicians so that men and women would have access to the best doctors in their area. You can visit our website www.SimplyAgeless411.com and ask these doctors questions and receive answers at no cost.

Male Menopause…It's Real

Sometimes called "puberty in reverse," male menopause - or
<u>andropause</u> as it is clinically diagnosed - is the period of a man's
life when production of a vital number of hormones - primarily
testosterone and thyroid hormones- begins to decline. Similarly,
women experience a reduction in estrogen and progesterone
production along with many other hormones during menopause.
But not everyone buys into the idea that males have their own
version of menopause. The public perception is that men of a
certain age are having "a mid-life crisis" that will eventually pass.

Decline usually begins in the 30s but becomes significant by
ages 45 – 60. Cases vary. There are men who remain virile into
their 80s with no visible signs of reduction in the hormone, but this
is extremely rare. In men, reduction of testosterone is typically a
gradual process that can take several years. Common symptoms of
andropause include a decrease in libido, erectile dysfunction,
muscle atrophy, weight gain and a decrease in lean body mass, a
general lack of energy, mood swings, depression, anxiety, and
memory loss. About 10 percent of men even experience hot
flashes. It's a serious medical condition that hasn't gotten the
attention it deserves. Gone untreated, male menopause can lead to
anemia and osteoporosis. It becomes evident from all these

possible symptoms that testosterone plays an extensive role in male health beyond just muscle building.

Dr. Stanton, one of our go-to experts on all things hormones, once again goes back to the simple blood test that can answer a myriad of questions and help you reboot your system. "Measuring testosterone levels through a blood test that can yield significant information," he says. "It is important to measure the bio-available testosterone in the body. Bound testosterone is ineffective because it is not available to the testosterone receptors throughout the body.

Thus, only bio-available testosterone will provide an accurate measurement." Dr. Stanton says the test isn't ordered as often as it should be - patients should be sure to ask their doctors about it, as it could make a powerful difference in quality of life. "Low levels of available testosterone are easily treated through a regimen of testosterone hormone weekly injections or daily gels and patches applied directly the skin," Dr. Stanton says. "For most men, the results are dramatic and immediate."

"While effective, testosterone replacement therapy should only be administered under strict medical supervision," he continues. "Physicians familiar with testosterone therapy know many tricks for optimizing results while at the same time minimizing side effects - such as those related to acne, estrogen conversion, and mood swings.

Candidates should first be screened for the prostate specific antigen (PSA), as prostate cancer can actually grow under testosterone therapy if the patient is predisposed. The therapy does not cause the cancer but it can exacerbate it if the condition already exists. Blood and liver enzyme levels also need to be monitored throughout the course of treatment." Dr. Stanton strongly advises that patients not self-medicate with over-the-counter 'natural' products that are often advertised in the back of men's magazines.

These supplements are not regulated by the FDA and can actually cause more harm than good. "Many of these products are pro-hormones that actually *convert* more frequently to estrogen than testosterone," he explains. "Real testosterone products are tightly regulated by the DEA and labeled as "Class III" controlled substances." Patients on Viagra or the like may also be candidates for testosterone therapy and the treatments can be prescribed simultaneously. Viagra does nothing to stimulate hormone production or the libido; it is only used to treat erectile dysfunction, which is different than low sex drive.

Exercise is a valuable tool in staving off depletion in testosterone. Exercise and working out actually stimulate production of testosterone in the body. Inactive men who gain considerable weight may have more estrogen in their bodies, since testosterone is converted into estrogen in the peripheral fat of the body if not 'burned off' through a regular course of exercise. Dr. Stanton reports that another contributor to "andropause" is low thyroid and adrenal function. "As much as 80 percent of the population (both men and women) have some degree of low thyroid function (hypothyroidism)," he says. "Even more unfortunate is the fact that this imbalance, which affects so many aspects of health, is frequently either misdiagnosed, misunderstood, or completely overlooked. For more on hypothyroidism, go back to Chapter 2 to review.

Whatever the case, there is an answer and a treatment. Women have benefited greatly from hormone therapy. Men deserve the same consideration to prolong quality of life.

Action Plan

for Hormone Replenishment

As we have discussed in this chapter, at approximately 25 years old we begin to age in very small steps, just like walking down a long flight of stairs. Growth hormone production begins to wane in our early 30s; by age 40, progesterone begins to decline and women begin to lose estrogen and men lose testosterone; then we both lose DHEA. The 30s and 40s are also the time when, after years of stressful living, the thyroid becomes sluggish and the adrenal glands become fatigued, leaving a person in a constant state of exhaustion.

The order of these losses as well as the timing will vary from one person to another. Yet the more we age, the more hormones we will lose. Our organs get to the point where they can no longer produce hormones on their own. Without supplementation, they can die and drag the others down with it. Until you begin to take bio-identical hormones, the entire cascade will continue. Your hormonal system can be reignited and the aging body can be resurrected. In this new age of integrative/anti-aging medicine you can take control of the aging process

We recommend bio-identical hormones because they are identical to the natural hormones that we are born with. We recommend that you work with a physician who specializes in bio-identical hormone replacement to get you started on your anti-aging journey. Here is a general guideline that will help you identify the phases of the anti-aging journey:

In Your 20s – This is the time to get a baseline hormonal profile so that you can identify the levels of all of your hormones when you are feeling your best. In your mid to late 20s begin taking preventative measures toward premature aging. Focus on maintaining a healthy lifestyle, keep your weight on track, workout four to five times a week (use weights three of those days), take a good multi-vitamin, fish oil and vitamin D. Starting early will increase the longevity of your hormones. For women, in the late 20s, estrogen levels begin to decline and supplementation may be needed.

In Your 30s - For both men and women, during the mid to late 30s you may begin to see a decline in the function of the thyroid, referred to as hypothyroidism and supplementation may be necessary. Growth Hormone is also on the decline but at this point can generally be stabilized with a high protein low carbohydrate diet along with three-four days a week of weight training. For women, the late 30s represent a time when some of the major hormones such as estrogen, progesterone, testosterone and DHEA will need supplementation. For men, the late 30s is the time that you may experience low testosterone and DHEA levels which may require supplementation. Nutritional supplements such as a multi-vitamin, fish oil, B vitamins and vitamin D should also be part of your anti-aging regimen to support your hormones.

In Your 40s - This is a critical phase for both men and women. Peri-menopause usually begins for women and andropause begins for men. This is the time to replenish major hormones and reverse the aging process with Growth Hormone, Testosterone, thyroid, cortisol (for adrenal function) estrogen, progesterone, DHEA and pregnenolone. Nutritional supplements such as a multi-vitamin, fish oil, B vitamins, vitamin D, vitamin C, CoQ10, Alpha Lipoic Acid and Resveratrol should also be part of your anti-aging regimen to support your hormones.

In Your 50s & beyond - This is the time to prepare for a new phase of your life, which is usually the happiest. Women usually are through menopause but many men are still going through andropause. If your blood profile indicates that you need hormonal supplementation, your hormone specialist will most likely recommend that you engage in the full spectrum of bio-identical hormone replacement including Growth Hormone, Testosterone, thyroid, cortisol (for adrenal function) estrogen, progesterone, DHEA and pregnenolone. Nutritional supplements such as a multi-vitamin, fish oil, B vitamins, vitamin D, vitamin C,

CoQ10, Alpha Lipoic Acid, Resveratrol, calcium and magnesium should also be part of your anti-aging regimen to support your hormones.

PART II a

Exploring the New World of Cosmetic Rejuvenation
Non-Surgical & Minimally Invasive Treatments

Chapter Four

Non-Surgical Cosmetic Treatments

In the next two chapters you will see that we have interviewed world class plastic surgeons and other medical professionals to bring you information on the latest cosmetic rejuvenation procedures available both surgically and without surgery. We have covered many popular procedures in the next two chapters, but for a more comprehensive list of all cosmetic surgery descriptions, costs and recovery times please visit our website at www.*SimplyAgeless411.com*.

We have had the privilege of meeting with these doctors you will meet in the next 2 chapters by attending medical conferences, listening to them speak, reading their weekly newsletters and sitting down with them for interviews. As you will see, they all have varying opinions on what works and what doesn't' work which, is a testament as to why, when choosing your own physician, you should thoroughly do your research and find a plastic surgeon, cosmetic surgeon, dermatologist or other medical professional who are board certified and/or are highly experienced in the procedure you are considering.

We are proud to present these fine doctors and interviews.

Making Grapes Out of Raisins

Non-surgical cosmetic procedures have become the "treatments of choice" for men and women around the world. Dermal fillers such as Restylane, Juvederm, Perlane, Radiesse, Sculptra and products such a Botox and Dysport along with a myriad of non-invasive laser treatments that are turning back the clock on the skin and changing the landscape of cosmetic medicine around the world.

We sat down with Dr. Bradley Friedman to explain this new phenomenon and to help provide insight into this new world of non-invasive cosmetic surgery. Voted as a "*Favorite Botox & Facial Filler Injection Doctor in Los Angeles,*" Dr. Bradley Friedman is highly skilled at administering aesthetic medicine including dermal fillers, Botox and laser treatments, he graduated from the Wake Forest University School of Medicine. His practice offers liquid facelifts, laser hair removal, laser vein treatments, Thermage, Eyes by Thermage, Cellulite by Thermage, ReFirme, IPL Fotofacial, Acne Laser, Facial and VStar laser treatments, many types of anti-aging and moisturizing facials.

__SimplyAgeless411:__ Thank you so much for taking the time to meet with us today, Dr. Friedman. In your opinion, which non-surgical procedure has the most dramatic effect on the facial features of men and women to help maintain a youthful appearance?

Dr. BF: Today in cosmetic medicine, the restoration of the cheek has become the treatment of choice for the aging face. As our faces age, the cheek fat pads diminish in size and drop in location. This causes our eyes to look older when the plump round "baby-cheek" does not frame the eye, giving a more hollow and sunken appearance.

When the shrinking cheek fat pads head south it also accentuates the smile lines, known as the nasolabial folds, creating a shadow in the fold that runs from the nose to lips. With advances in dermal fillers this age related loss of volume can be corrected and the youthful face can be restored. This is like taking raisins and making grapes out of them.

When I started using collagen to plump and restore lips in 1996, the treatments typically lasted 3 to 4 months. New soft-tissue fillers like Restylane, Juvederm and Radiesse last 6 - 24 months, depending on individual factors like motion, metabolism and location of treatment. For example, when I fill earlobes, which shrink and prune with age, fillers typically last a lot longer than the same filler in the lip. We all move our lips more than our earlobes and these motions can break up the fillers more rapidly, but in combination with Botox in selected areas, I aid in relaxing the muscles that advance the breakdown of fillers.

Restylane, Perlane & Juvederm has become the most popular fillers for lips. They contain a natural component that keeps water in the skin by binding water and plumping skin and lips. These sugar fillers are made from hyaluronic acid and are longer lasting than bovine collagen; their gel like texture passes the "kiss test" and highlights a very natural shape in the lips. We all lose lip volume as we age, and the lips shrink, invert and wrinkle. A little bit of "resty" (Restylane) fixes this and makes the lips look younger, plump and kissable. Give yourself 3-5 days to recover from this as the lips are very vascular and bruising can occur.

SimplyAgeless411: Are these procedures painful or are they well tolerated by most patients?

Dr. BF: My patients rarely bruise due to the anatomical differences. Best news of all- it doesn't hurt. Radiesse, a calcium based dermal filler, is ideal in the cheek area. Radiesse lifts and fills out the face for more youthful contours and effectively decreases the visible nasolabial fold (smile line) to give you more to smile about. By *artistically* re-volumizing the cheek area, the eyes look younger and loose skin is replenished.

Fillers are better than a face lift because there is no scarring, no risk of general anesthesia, little down time, and a more *natural* appearance! The entire experience takes about 20 minutes after a topical anesthetic is applied for your comfort, and please allow 1-2 days for swelling in this area to go down. The end result is a younger, softer, well rested version of youth.

SimplyAgeless411: Wow…times have certainly changed in the last few years! Simply putting the volume back that diminishes with age seems like such an easy way to restore the youthful appearances of the face. Do you find that both men and women are having these procedures done?

Dr. B.F.: Oh yes, definitely! These days I have just as many male patients coming in as female patients for dermal fillers, Botox, lasers for the skin and hair removal. In the world we live in both men and women really care about looking good and staying youthful for as long as possible.

SimplyAgeless411: I know exactly what you mean, Dr. Friedman, we believe that our society is changing dynamically. Both men and women are realizing that by making just a few hormonal changes and cosmetic tweaks in their twenties, thirties and forties, they can maintain a youthful appearance throughout their entire lives. Gone are the days of the average person entering their forties and fifties looking haggard and old and subsequently feeling old. Sadly, many people spend a lot of time and energy pining for and remembering the days of their youth. Life really just begins getting fun and interesting when you enter your forties and there is so much to look forward to. Thank you so much, Dr. Friedman, for all that you do to help people look and feel better about themselves. We really appreciate the time you spent with us today!

Liquid Facelifts – Do You Have Skull Face?

To continue our research into non-invasive cosmetic treatments we sat down with Dr. Lisa Cassileth to get her thoughts on the new non-invasive procedures. Dr. Cassileth is a plastic and reconstructive surgeon certified by the American Board of Plastic Surgery. She specializes in facelifts, tummy tucks, rhinoplasty, blepharoplasty (eyes), breast augmentation, body contouring, laser treatments and facial fillers. She has been featured on *Dr. 90210, Rachael Ray, Entertainment Tonight and The Discovery Channel.* In addition to her main practice in Beverly Hills, she just opened a medical clinic, CassilethMueller Cosmetic Medicine, focusing on cosmetic medicine with the latest technology in facial fillers and a myriad of laser treatments for the skin and body.

SimplyAgeless411:   Hello Dr. Cassileth and thank you so much for giving us a few moments of your time to discuss new trends in cosmetic medicine, more specifically the more non-invasive procedures that area now available. What are your thoughts on non-surgical facelifts?

Dr. LC: Your cheeks have jowls. Your chin has marionette lines. Your face is... drooping! Does this mean you need a facelift? Has the time really come for you to get a facelift?

Expensive, traditional facelifts alone can be a big mistake for a certain type of face. Tightly pulled skin stretched over cheekbones doesn't just look unnatural and plastic surgery-ized; it looks old! In many cases women and their plastic surgeons are missing the boat. Or really, they are missing the fat. What is lacking is the contour of youth.

Look at your old photos and notice: the rounded cheeks; the temples are flat, not hollowed; the fullness of the jaw line. These are important indicators of a youthful face. When this fat is gone, the face sags, and no matter how tightly the skin is pulled in a facelift, your face will not recover its youthfulness. A liquid facelift may instead be the ideal solution for you.

SimplyAgeless411: So what is the liquid facelift?

Dr. LC: It is the injection of fillers into the face to restore the contour of youth. In fact, many signs of aging - for example, jowls, downturned lips, hollowed eyes, and overly visible bony contours (aka "skull face") - can be completely reversed. A variety of products can be used, from hyaluronic acids, like Juvederm™ and Restylane®, to Radiesse®, to my personal favorite, Sculptra™, which lasts years longer than the other products and builds your own collagen over time.

__SimplyAgeless411__: So how does the liquid facelift work?

Dr. LC: Typically, when using Sculptra, the product is injected in several sessions, so that the change is gradual. The best candidates are men and women without much fat on their faces who have facial sagging. If Sculptra™ is used; the product costs about $800 per session (depending on how much product is used) and usually takes about three sessions for the best results.

__SimplyAgeless411__: We know that you are on a tight schedule this morning and we are very grateful for the time and great information that you have shared with us. I think we are all a little relieved that there are so many new non-surgical options that will refresh our appearance are now available to us.

Laser Treatments...Fraxel, Fractional, Co2, Erbium – Which One Is Best?

There is a lot of buzz going around about which laser works the best...which one goes the deepest and which ones cause the most down time. We sat down with Dr. Edward Jonas Domanskis and asked him to give us the 411 on laser treatments and to tell us everything that we need to know...and he did that and much more!

Dr. Edward Domanskis is a board certified plastic surgeon located in Orange County, California. His expertise is in body contouring, facial surgery and minimally invasive surgery. He introduced his highly acclaimed "**Minicision lift**" on *Good Morning America* and he also completed a Cosmetic Surgery Video Series which is sold nationwide.

SimplyAgeless411*:* Hello Dr. Domanskis, let me first say how grateful we are to you for meeting with us today to discuss various laser treatments that are currently available. We are excited to learn as much as you can teach us about the latest advancements in laser technology.

Dr. ED: The use of lasers to treat facial problems is a relatively new procedure. Many different lasers have been, and are being developed to treat specific conditions. They can be roughly grouped into two categories depending on their wavelength, i.e. ones that target specific types of cells, like hemoglobin in blood vessels (pulse dye laser) and those that are ablative, that just vaporize everything they are focused at, like the erbium and carbon dioxide lasers (CO_2).

SimplyAgeless411: So the Erbium and the CO_2 are the ones that most plastic surgeons and dermatologists use for resurfacing the skin, correct?

Dr. ED: Yes, the Erbium and the CO_2 are the types primarily used in facial rejuvenation. The depth and extent of vaporization is controlled by various modalities, like the length of time that the laser is focused on an area, the size of the spot that comes out of the laser machine as well as the laser's power setting and frequency of the pulses emitted.

The smaller the spot size, the lower the power output and the longer it is focused on an area as well as how many times it is passed over the same area determines the amount of surface tissue it will remove and damage to the surrounding tissues it will cause.

Essentially, a burn is produced which may be superficial (1st degree) down to a deep or 3rd degree. The depth of the burn will determine how long it will take to heal. A superficial ablation or burn of the skin surface by the laser will produce some redness or inflammation and take a few days to go away. The deeper 2nd degree level will cause some blistering, scabbing as well as redness (inflammation) which should still heal within a two week period.

The latter though may persist for several months until it heals. If the depth of penetration of the laser causes a 3rd degree burn, then scarring would result.

Facial resurfacing with the CO2 laser became extremely popular because it was very effective in rejuvenating the skin, helping to reverse primarily the textural changes associated with aging, sun damage, and smoking. This laser almost totally replaced dermabrasion in the treatment of acne scarring. When properly used, the complications were minimal, but used incorrectly could be disastrous creating extensive scarring. The side-effects, such as prolonged redness (average of four months with limited sun-exposure) and difference in coloring from treated and non-treated areas became more troublesome. Both of these usually faded with time but others were left with whiter faces (caused by the removal of any existing tan which is confined to the outermost layers of skin) redundant creepiness and uneven coloration of the neck. Also, because only the face has "thick" skin, treatment was limited to this area. If these conditions were acceptable, the results of the treatment of the face could be quite dramatic!

To minimize these side-effects, a "gentler" laser, the erbium (often referred to as "Fraxel"), was introduced for facial resurfacing. This increased the margin of safety, decreased the side-effects, and length of healing, but also compromised the results. The Erbium does not penetrate as deeply as the CO2 laser.

It takes about five passes of the Erbium laser to equal one of the CO_2 laser! The Erbium laser treatment, however, no longer required an anesthetic but could be done with a topical ointment.

The next major advance was the introduction of a fractionated laser, first the Fractionated Erbium and then the Fractionated CO_2 laser. Essentially a grid is placed on the opening of the laser which blocks a portion of the beam that is emitted by the laser. So, instead of a whole area that is treated, the shutter effect limits the burned area by the laser to a certain percentage (about 50% plus) only to be ablated or burned. This limits the burn which limits the pain and also allows treatment with only a topical anesthetic.

The untreated remaining skin suffers less damage/burn resulting in less inflammation (redness), usually minimal blistering and scabbing and a shorter time of healing. On average this is between one to two weeks with minimal, if any, redness persisting. Also, there is less of a need to protect oneself from the sun to prevent post-treatment color changes (hyper-pigmentation). Finally, and quite significantly, other areas besides the face, like the neck, chest or even hands can be treated.

Because of the above benefits, the Fractionated CO_2 laser has become the instrument of choice for most plastic surgeons and dermatologists in treating sun-damaged, aging and smokers' skin that show textural changes. The Fractionated Erbium laser, just like its predecessor requires many more passes or several treatments to achieve the results of the Fractionated CO_2 laser.

SimplyAgeless411: Do any of these lasers actually tighten the skin on the face or neck?

Dr. ED: Contrary to popular belief, neither laser causes more than a temporary skin tightening. The laser world has evolved and improved in its quest for the most effective treatment with the least amount of side-effects or complications. The guidance of your plastic surgeon or dermatologist is still important to achieve the best possible improvement for your level of skin damage.

SimplyAgeless411: Thank you so much for this in-depth look at the evolution and benefits of laser resurfacing of the skin. Our mission is to help people navigate their way through all of the new technologies available to help them to achieve the best possible results.

Major Breakthroughs in Vein Removal

Some major breakthroughs are happening in the world of vein removal and we wanted to be first on the scene to get the news. We sat down with Dr. Wayne Gradman, who is located right here in the heart of Beverly Hills, to discuss the latest developments.

Dr. Gradman is one of the most prominent vein removal experts in the world.

He graduated from Harvard Medical School and received postgraduate vascular training at UCLA Medical Center and Cedars-Sinai Medical Center. He is board certified in Phlebology, Vascular Surgery, and General Surgery. For many years, Dr. Gradman, practiced vascular surgery at the world renowned Cedars-Sinai Medical Center located in Los Angeles. He is a member American College of Phlebology, which focuses on the treatment of varicose vein problems, and the American Venous Forum, the nation's most prestigious organization dedicated to the study of venous disorders.

SimplyAgeless411*:* Vein removal is such a fascinating subject and we feel honored to speak with you, Dr. Gradman, about the latest advancements in this field. You know…unsightly veins can make a person look much older than they are but most people think of varicose veins or spider veins on the legs as the only area of the body where veins are treated for cosmetic reasons. Can you tell us what other areas can be treated successfully?

Dr. G: Leg vein procedures are the most popular; however, I also treat veins on the back of the hands, the face and on the chest! In fact, I am one of the few physicians that know how to successfully treat varicose veins on the face.

SimplyAgeless411: Isn't treating facial veins dangerous? Does it leave a scar? How do you treat them?

Dr. G: No, treating facial veins the way I treat them is very safe and effective. Minimal bruising, then a period where the bruise may turn a brownish color and then it fades…and the vein is gone! Many women try to hide the bulging veins on their temples by wearing bangs, even if they would rather show their entire face. I inject facial veins with my special foamed solution. No, it does not leave a scar and patients are thrilled with the results.

SimplyAgeless411: Why would a person need their chest treated for unsightly veins?

Dr. G: I have had many female patients that have had breast augmentation. After the procedure, for some reason, they can see big veins on their chest on the top of their breasts. They feel very upset that they still don't have a nice cleavage area after undergoing corrective breast surgery. So they come to me to treat their chest veins, which I do and the result is terrific.

SimplyAgeless411: What about hands? I would think that every woman who is over 35 and has bulging veins on the back of her hands would want to have them corrected. Yet, it seems that most women are not aware that this is an option available to them or think that it's dangerous to close those veins. Please explain.

Dr. G: It's true that most women are not aware of how quickly and easily the veins on the back of their hands can be treated and improved. Phlebology is a relatively new field and hasn't gotten the attention yet that it deserves. Many women who have heard of the procedure are afraid that they will lose circulation in their hands if they have the bulging veins treated. This is not true. The body does not need the surface veins in order to function properly. What are important are the veins that are deeper inside of the body. We do not treat those for aesthetic reasons, only surface veins that are unsightly.

SimplyAgeless411: You are a Phlebologist, a physician that specializes in the treatment of veins. Is the practice of Phlebology recognized by the American Medical Association as a legitimate field of medicine?

Dr. G: Yes. The AMA and other medical groups recently acknowledged that Phlebology is a real specialty. I believe this is due to the tremendous advances that have been made in the treatment of both cosmetic and serious vein conditions in the last 15-20 years.

SimplyAgeless411: Up until 5-10 years ago, people used to go to surgeons to get their varicose veins stripped in the hospital. The procedure sounded very painful and terribly invasive. Would you tell us about this?

Dr. G: People who had varicose veins used to get their veins stripped in a hospital. This required general anesthesia, a one week stay in the hospital (on average), pain, major bruising, swelling and big scars. Because of this, I believe many people did not get their varicose veins treated and lived with the discomfort, achiness, and disfigurement of their legs.

SimplyAgeless411:   How do modern day phlebologists (vein disorder physicians) treat varicose veins now?

Dr. G: First of all, we do not need to strip the leaky saphenous veins (which are usually deeper veins one can not see that is causing the problem) or the more surface varicose veins that are visual. For the deeper veins, the treatment is now minimally invasive and requires no anesthesia. We use either a laser (which was developed in Europe) or radio frequency for larger veins (which was developed in the U.S.). I always use my in-office ultrasound to properly diagnose the deeper veins that can not be seen with the naked eye, called the saphenous veins.

If a patient has leaky saphenous veins, they must be treated first or the surface problematic veins will not respond well to treatment. I must treat the medical issue first and then address the cosmetic portion. I use the ultrasound during treatment to assure accuracy. Patients are very appreciative of not having to get an ultrasound done in a radiology office. This saves them time and money.

SimplyAgeless411: Do you ever surgically remove the smaller varicose veins?

Dr. G: Yes, we do. However, the procedure is performed with only local anesthesia and in most cases, leaves no scars. We make tiny incisions on both sides of the surface vein and remove them. The incisions close up naturally and do not require stitches. They heal very fast with minimal bruising.

SimplyAgeless411: Is it true that you oftentimes opt to inject the smaller varicose veins, rather than remove them surgically? If so, can you explain the procedure?

Dr. G: I like to use a foamed solution that has Sotradecol in it. I have created a special foamed formulation that I have used to inject inside the surface varicose veins and then compress them. The FDA has not approved this solution yet for the use on larger veins. However, I have had tremendous success with this product as it leaves no scars, works very well and has a high degree of patient satisfaction.

SimplyAgeless411: The most well-known vein procedure for treating spider veins is schlerotherapy. What is that and how is it performed?

Dr. G: Schlerotherapy is the injection of small spider veins with a liquid solution: typically either a saline solution or FDA approved Sotradecol. The vein is injected and then collapses. The blood is then reabsorbed into the body and the vein disappears. Is takes the typical patient about 4-6 weeks for the vein and/or bruising to heal. This requires no anesthesia and is mildly uncomfortable with brief stinging for a moment. The patient can resume normal activity immediately.

SimplyAgelss411: You do not like to use saline, although many dermatologists use it. What is the reason you prefer Sotradecol to saline?

Dr. G: Saline hurts and has more staining. By staining I mean it tends to leave a mark on the skin. Saline does not usually yield consistently good results. Sotradecol, on the other hand, is very effective and only mildly uncomfortable and does not tend to stain. It works by irritating the vein and closing it faster. In my opinion, it is far superior.

SimplyAgeless411: Aside from Sotradecol, is there any other product that is used to treat spider veins successfully? If so, what is it and do you like it?

Dr. G: The newest injectable for spider veins is Polidocanol. I have tried it, but I still prefer Sotradecol. I am completely satisfied with Sotradecol and do not feel the need to use anything else at this time.

SimplyAgeless411: Dermatologists use lasers to treat facial veins. You prefer to inject facial veins. What is the reason?

Dr. G: Facial veins that are bigger blue veins, above the eyebrows, the temporal area, and under the eyes do not respond well to laser. That's why I inject them with a foamed solution. I get very good results.

SimplyAgeless411: What about those tiny broken capillaries on the face such as around and on the nose, and on the cheeks and chin. How are those best treated?

Dr. G: Years ago, these small veins were treated with an electric needle that cauterized them. Then they scabbed for about a week and then healed. While the procedure was effective, too many patients experienced scarring. So doctors, mostly dermatologists switched to lasers. However, most lasers require 3 treatments and don't always do a good job at solving the problem.

A new laser called Veinwave has just been introduced. It is a laser that works like an electric needle without scarring the patient. It seems to give superior results.

SimplyAgeless411: How much of your practice is devoted to cosmetic vein procedures and how much is actual medical issues?

Dr. G: Seventy-five percent of my practice is cosmetic and twenty-five percent is medical.

SimplyAgeless411: When you say "medical vein issues" what are you referring to?

Dr. G: There is a large segment of our population that suffers from leg ulcers, which are very painful and horribly unsightly. Physicians used to think that these leg ulcers were caused by phlebitis. Many people could not be helped. I have found that more than half of these patients are being treated successfully by performing cosmetic vein removal as I do with my varicose vein patients. I am able to use my in-office ultrasound machine to treat and diagnose effectively. I use my foamed solution to inject the vein directly under the ulcer. Then the ulcer heals up beautifully. Almost all leg ulcers can be treated and/or cured.

SimplyAgeless411: It sounds like there are no reasons why a person should suffer with unsightly varicose veins, spider veins or painful leg ulcers, if they can afford to correct them. For actual medical vein procedures, do insurance companies cover them?

Dr. G: Many of the medical vein procedures I perform are covered by medical insurance. However, those that are purely cosmetic are most often not covered.

SimplyAgeless411: This has been such an incredibly enlightening interview, Dr. Gradman; we are so excited to be able to share this information with all of our readers. There are many people who suffer from diabetes that get leg ulcers and usually the first thing their doctors will want to do is a skin graft. Treating the vein underneath the leg ulcer makes so much more sense and it's this kind of "under the radar" information that keeps us doing what we do here at SimplyAgeless411.

People are at the mercy of the training that their physicians may or may not decide to take. We have discovered that across the board if you have a health issue, doctors will treat differently depending on their level of expertise. It is up to the patient to empower themselves with as much research as possible on both the illness that they have and the doctor that they select. Most doctors have a database of approximately 25,000 patients, and many do not have the time or energy to learn about the latest advancements and treatments for every illness or new procedure.

Rejuvenating Dry, Itchy Eyes

While we don't normally think of rejuvenating dry, itchy eyes as a non-surgical cosmetic treatment, having scratchy bloodshot eyes can certainly be aging to your appearance and we wanted to know how to treat them.

We contacted one of American's top Ophthalmologists', Cynthia Boxrud MD, FACS, who is a medical specialist in Facial Ophthalmic, Plastic and Reconstructive Surgery, as well as Orbital and Ophthalmic Oncology. She is one of 4 % of female surgeons in the United States that holds two "fellowships"; medicine's most advanced formal training. Dr. Boxrud has been elected by her peers into *America's Top Doctors, America's Top Ophthalmologists and America's Top Cosmetic Surgeons* from 2001 until present and America's Top Doctor's for Cancer in 2005. Dr. Boxrud was happy to give us her top 3 remedies:

1) **Flax Seed Oil or Omega 3-6-9 -** Take Flax Seed Oil or Omega 3-6-9. One tablet a day. There has been some evidence that taken orally, these supplements help change the oil in the glands around the eyes.

2)   **Drink Alkaline Water** - Drinking alkaline water or water
with electrolytes (Smart Water). There is no anecdotal evidence
but I have had great success with patients.

3)   **Artificial Tears** - Using artificial tears without preservatives
four times a day. Remember, "Water the grass when it's green not
when it's brown". Lubricate your eyes when you are without
symptoms of dryness. Thank you Dr. Boxrud! We appreciate
your insightful advice!

Facial Fillers vs. Fat Transfer: Which Procedure is Best?

Some doctors recommend fat transfers as facial fillers to fill
out wrinkles and improve hollowness in the face while many
doctors recommend using facial fillers such as Juvederm, Sculptra,
Radiesse or Restylane for the same problem. We met up with Dr.
Rady Rahban, a board certified plastic surgeon in Beverly Hills
who studied and worked closely with Dr. Garth Fisher, the world
renowned plastic surgeon featured on the hit ABC television show
Extreme Makeover to weigh-in on which procedure works the best.

SimplyAgeless411: Thanks so much for meeting with us today. I
think everyone is a little confused about which dermal fillers work
the best—temporary or permanent. Can you provide us with a little

background on these procedures and give us your thoughts on which ones might work the best?

Dr. RR: This is a very common question... it can be a bit confusing. Essentially, as we age we lose volume or the fullness in our face. It turns out that this is as important, if not more important, than the excess skin we develop. We need to fill in the areas that have lost volume, such as the cheeks, but with what? Once you determine that filler is needed to treat the face, you should decide what is going to work best for you.

Today, there a numerous options and each have its own pro's and con's. Simply stated, fillers can be divided into permanent and temporary fillers. Most patients today tend to use temporary fillers such as Restylane or Juvederm. They are safe, well-studied, most have limited side effects and good results when injected by a skilled practitioner.

Most importantly, they are temporary, so if there is an error or you as the patient are unhappy with the result, the good news is that it will eventually dissolve and you find a solution that gives you the look you want. This advantage is also a disadvantage because it *is* temporary; you'll need to come back after about six months or so to get the same treatment. Patients want their desired look to last forever and not have to undergo the procedure again and again.

Okay, this leads me to fat injections. Fat is considered permanent filler. It's harvested from the patient's own body and carefully transferred to areas that need volume replacement, or "plumping." Sounds great, right? However, there are many things to consider with fat that need to be understood prior to jumping on the table. First of all, fat transfer is usually not a one-time procedure but will require two to three visits for the desired results, because all of the fat that is harvested at the first visit does not survive the transfer and the initial satisfying results tend to fade with time. So, here again, repeated rounds of the treatment are needed to maintain the look.

Secondly, fat transfer is much more unpredictable than temporary filler such as Juvederm. We never know how much fat will survive and on which side of the face....so be careful. If a mistake is made, poor judgment is used by an inexperienced practitioner or you just don't like the final results, removing the injected fat it is an incredibly difficult process, though not impossible.

Finally, the recovery time for this procedure is much longer than with temporary fillers because of the harvesting and application elsewhere, it is something of a minor surgery procedure. It is more expensive in the short run, although in long-run it will save you much more money.

I'd say for the patient new to fillers or one that does not want the hassle of long recoveries and potential risks, stick to temporary fillers. For patients that are more tolerant of risks and wish for a longer and often more natural result, then fat grafting is an excellent option. Know what you're getting into, weigh each of the options available, and decide what's right for you. My best advice is that it should be done by a trained practitioner who has experience and a strong rate of success.

SimplyAgeless411: Thank you, Dr. Rahban, for "filling" us in what options are available. Your time is much appreciated!

New Treatments for the Aging Neck

As we get older, gravity catches up with all of us. And while we've maybe had the fine lines and wrinkles on our face treated by one method or another, the neck sometimes goes untouched, until you realize the sagging is starting to look like a "waddle". We sat down once again with our friend, Dr. Edward Domanskis, to learn about the exciting new treatments and procedures that can make dramatic improvements to the aging neck.

Dr. Domanskis is a Board Certified Plastic Surgeon located in Orange County, California. His expertise is in body contouring, facial surgery and minimally invasive surgery. He introduced his highly acclaimed "Minicision lift" on *Good Morning America* and he also completed a Cosmetic Surgery Video Series which is sold nationwide.

__SimplyAgeless411__: Good morning, Dr. Domanskis, thank you for meeting with us today to discuss new procedures for the aging neck. If there is one area that both men and women are equally sensitive about, it's the way their neck ages. Tell us about the latest procedures that can help.

Dr. ED: It's true, as we age, things begin to sag. The neck is no exception. You'll at first notice a small fullness just under the chin as early as in your 20s, which can progress to a "turkey gobbler" appearance later in life. This inevitable progression is affected by genetics (how your parents aged) as well as weight loss. This descent can be forestalled and even eliminated by various procedures.

The initial fullness you see can be treated by liposuction, even under a local anesthetic as an outpatient. It takes a short time to perform through a tiny puncture mark just below the chin. Bruising is minimal and dressings may not even be necessary. Removal of this relatively small amount of fat, which acts as a weight on the tissues and pulls them down, may result in significant less neck sag at a later age.

Tightening the neck and reducing the excess skin non-surgically can be achieved with radiofrequency waves (as with *Thermage* and *Titan*). They literally burn the collagen under the skin surface, which causes a contraction of the tissues so that new collagen is generated. Most patients get satisfying results, which lasts an average of two years. The long-lasting effects are nothing like what can be achieved with a neck lift.

Some "quick fixes" would include a small cut below the chin to remove a small amount of excess skin only. Here, the width of the scar is limited by the wideness of the chin area. If more neck sag is present, a neck lift would be necessary, with the scars hidden behind the ears and extending along or into the hairline. This produces a clean, sharper profile. Think of it as the bottom half of a traditional facelift. Those unsightly cords, which are bands of a vestigial muscle called the platysma, can be minimized during the procedure, but don't be surprised if they return some years later.

Botox can be injected into the platysma bands for some improvement to prevent the bands from becoming more prominent but it does not eliminate them. These cosmetic procedures treat the sagginess of the neck they do not address the textural changes like creppiness, which is unevenness of the actual skin surface because of a loss of collagen.

Think of an older person you know whose skin seemed thin and frail, like crepe paper. This is primarily caused by sun damage over the years, and can be exacerbated by smoking. The best treatment is definitely prevention, meaning either stay out of the sun or protect use sunscreens and, of course, *do not smoke.* Creams can help but only to a certain extent.

Some people have rings around their neck, sometimes called the "permanent necklace" that they've had since their 20s. Injectable fillers like Restylane will fill them out; however, a Fractionated CO2 laser and/or Thermage would be the best course of treatment. (Find useful information on laser/thermage earlier in this book)

A recent and significant advancement in treating this area is with the Fractionated CO2 laser, which "burns" off the top, dead, aged, sun-damaged skin layers. Besides the neck, the laser can be used to treat the chest or décolletage area also. In less than one hour as an outpatient, this treatment can reverse the years of exposure to the sun and give you back a smoother, less wrinkled neck which you will forever meticulously guard. This procedure can be done with a topical anesthetic. Healing takes an average of about 10 days and this procedure can be repeated until the desired improvement is achieved.

SimplyAgeless411: This is fantastic news for the many men and women who have been looking for a non-surgical way to tighten up their neck area. Thank you so much for taking the time to visit with us today!

Turning Back the Hands of Time *on Your Hands*

The hands are one of the first areas of the body, after the face, to show the visible signs of aging. They are also one of the first things that people notice about you, after the face. With time and exposure, the hands may lose fat which can result in a thin, transparent, bony or "creppey" appearance, much like the skin in the neck, as discussed in the previous section. The veins and tendons may become more visible, and pigmentation problems such as age spots may develop.

Fortunately, according to top dermatologists and plastic surgeons, hand rejuvenation procedures can restore a smoother, more youthful appearance. According to several of the plastic surgeons and dermatologists that we have interviewed, hand rejuvenation can be achieved with a variety of different procedures, either performed on their own or in combination. Good candidates for treatment include healthy individuals who have realistic expectations for improving the appearance of their hands.

For thin, transparent-looking hands resulting from a loss of fat, doctors often use Radiesse. This injectable filler can be administered in an office setting using a local anesthetic. A single treatment (1 syringe @ approximately $800) provides instant results that can last anywhere from 12 to 18 months. Results may vary, so depending on the amount of fat loss in your hands, two or three treatments may be required for optimal results. While treatment is relatively painless and normal activities can be resumed immediately, some patients may experience minor bruising or swelling. Other injectable fillers may also be used for hand rejuvenation including Sculptra, Restylane and Juvederm.

Thermage is a good option for treating loose, "creppey" skin on the hands. It uses non-invasive radio frequency waves to heat the deep layers of the skin, tightening it and promoting new collagen growth. Treatment is done in the doctor's office with an oral medication to minimize discomfort. There is no downtime after the procedure; you can go back to your normal routine right away. You'll see results immediately, and continued improvement as collagen growth increases. Cost: Approximately $1200.

Laser resurfacing is an ideal treatment for age spots and other pigmentation problems occurring on the hands. The laser can also help thicken the skin of the hands as the heat encourages new collagen growth. There is minimal downtime, though some flaking of the skin may occur. Final results are apparent after three to six months. Cost: Approximately $1500.

There are several other procedures for turning back time on your hands. ***LipoStructure*** removes fat from one area of the body (usually the belly or hips) and transfers it into the hands to smooth them out. Cost: Approximately $2,000

Chemical peels may be used to treat age spots and other pigmentation problems, and ***Sclerotherapy*** can help to diminish the appearance of unsightly veins (more details on this in our previous discussion with Dr. Gradman a few pages back)

Lip Augmentation: Lip Lifts, Enhancements & Earlobe Rejuvenation

Lip injections are the only way for men and women to perk up that beautiful smile. That's right guys, we have the 411 that many men out there are also having their "lips done."

We connected with Dr. Domanskis again to find out more about Lip-lifts, Lip-reductions and more.

SimplyAgeless411: Dr. Domanskis, once again, thank you for taking time to speak with us again. This time, we're seeking your professional advice on the lip procedures that are available. What's happening in the world of lip augmentation?

Dr. ED: Yes, of course, I am happy to answer any questions that you have. The upper **Liplift** is a procedure that elevates the position of the upper lip with respect to the teeth, to give a broader smile. The amount of pink lip that is seen is also increased, giving the patient wider lips.

The lips can also be made fuller with implants or by injecting fillers or abdominal fat into the lips at the same surgical session. The overall effect of the **Liplift** is a more aesthetically pleasing mouth and a younger appearance. The patient satisfaction rate is very high.

In our youth, the lips are fuller and poutier. The pink part of the lip can be 1/3 to 1/2 the volume of the moustache area in general. Some of us are born with naturally long upper lips. This procedure is designed to shorten the upper lip, which allows people even in their 20s to benefit.

As we age, all the bones of the body (including the face) retract and diminish, causing the flesh of the face to "hang" more. The soft tissue and fat of the face atrophy so the skin itself also falls. The older upper lip is characterized by a thin or non-existent vermilion (the pink part) and a smile that does not show the teeth. The *Liplift* can correct this.

There are many options today to improve our lips and enhance our natural smiles. A *Liplift-nasal* removes a strip of skin below the nose to produce the desired height the patient wants the upper lip to be. Because there is an incision, a small scar is left above the lip line, but the healing time is quick and successful. This particular procedure is usually performed on women, who can cover a tiny scar with lipstick. Different fillers like Fascia, and Advanta implants can be placed at the same time as the Liplift-nasal to give more fullness to the lips. A **V to Y** advancement of the tissue from the inside of the lips can be done to gain more fullness without adding any fillers. Patients can "customize" they way they want their lips to look, which many find empowering.

All of these procedures can be done as an outpatient with a local anesthetic in the office. Most take a little over an hour to complete. All external sutures are taken out the next day. There will be some tenderness for the first couple of days. After two weeks, swelling and bruising will go away and you'll be left with full, beautiful lips.

Fees for procedures like these vary, but in general, the patient can expect to spend between $2,500 and $6,000.

SimplyAgeless411: We also understand that many people are unhappy about having lips that are too large. Can you tell us about the Lip Reduction?

Dr. ED: A **Lip Reduction** can usually be performed as an outpatient and even under local anesthesia in the office. A strip of tissue is removed between the inside and outside the mouth so the scar heals the best and is minimally visible. No dressings can be placed, so patients should expect to limit their activities and avoid frequent talking for at least one week. The swelling is maximal at that time, but usually goes down to an acceptable level within two weeks. The lips may not fully heal for several months, though. A lip reduction can be performed on both the upper and lower lips. The cost of each is about $3000-4000.

SimplyAgeless411: It's great to know that there is a solution to almost every aesthetic problem. What can you tell us about the new "earlobe regeneration" procedure we've been hearing so much about lately?

Dr. ED: Certainly. **Earlobe Rejuvenation** is growing in popularity as it becomes more mainstream. The earlobes are made of soft skin and a small amount of fatty tissue. The size and shape vary from person to person, as we've all noticed among our friends and family. Like fingerprints, each set of earlobes is different. Earlobes generally become larger and longer with age and they begin to sag. A large earlobe may require substantial ear jewelry for appropriate balance; small studs may appear "lost" within the space of a fleshy earlobe. Large earlobes can be sagging and hang down too far, which can be corrected by decreasing the excess curvature. Some earlobes appear rather "fleshy" and elongated, but this too can easily be corrected.

I include an earlobe reduction in almost every facelift that I do in both men and women. More and more, I am also performing many earlobe reductions apart from facelifts. I simply remove the lower "saggy" part and round out the lobe that has stretched out and elongated. When earrings have torn through the earlobe, I freshen the edges and re-suture the split. The earlobes can be re-pierced after several weeks, but in a slightly different location or the tear can recur. Scars on the earlobes heal quite well and are barely noticeable. Any sort of earlobe enhancement is done under local anesthesia and is minimally invasive. In most cases, the procedure takes less than an hour. The cost is approximately $2,200.

SimplyAgeless411: What non-surgical techniques are available to restore and correct earlobes?

Dr ED: Non-surgical options are available, including injectable dermal fillers such as Juvederm, Restylane and Radiesse to plump out sagging earlobes. The effects can last up to a year. Thermage and laser resurfacing may also be used to tighten the skin, however, they are very limited in their effects on the ears.

SimplyAgeless411: As always, thanks so much for your time today, Dr. Domanskis.

Skin Tighteners, Radiofrequency & Infrared Technology

We interviewed several doctors on the topic of the latest advancements in Skin Tighteners, radiofrequency and Infrared Light technologies, which can tighten, tone, firm and soften the skin. Currently, brands such as Thermage, Accent, Titan, SkinTyte and Vela-Smooth are the market leaders. Interestingly enough, we discovered that a large number of doctors support and endorse these technologies and believe they are the next best thing, however, an equally large number of doctors believe that the benefits of these new technologies are only temporary and offer little overall improvements. So, at least for now, the professional verdict is still out. Let us take a deeper look into some of these new technologies and let you, the consumer be the judge.

Overall, skin tighteners can prompt new collagen to form, by the use of Thermal (heat) energy that is delivered beneath the skin to safely injure the dermis. An inflammatory response is initiated, which stimulates the activity of fibroblasts to create more collagen.

Collagen acts like a scaffolding or a firm foundation for the skin. However, as the skin ages and the body goes through dramatic changes like weight loss, weigh gain and pregnancy, the skin's foundation begins to crumble and the quality and amount of collagen become poor. That's where skin-tightening treatments come in. These new technologies can help create thick, strong, plump collagen inside so that the skin on the outside looks smooth and refined. These devices are targeting strictly at tightening the skin without damaging the outer layer of skin so that there is no downtime.

How These Skin Tightening Devices Work – The Procedure

These treatments are non-invasive radiofrequency energy which are electric and magnetic energy coupled with radio waves. They emit short yet intense pulses to oscillate through the skin and deliver heat to the deepest layer of the skin at low temperatures without damaging the outer layer of skin.

These devices can be used on many areas of the body such as the face, neck, arms, stomach, buttocks and thighs. First, the skin is cooled with a built-in plate to prevent burning. The cooling plate is removed and then the heat plate is quickly applied to a targeted area of the body emitting energy deep into the cells to create collagen. A few moments later the skin is then cooled again to prevent burning. The deepest layers of the skin react to the heat causing a slight injury and inflammation that signals the existing collagen to contract and causes new collagen to be made over the next 90 days.

Most doctors recommend these treatments for men and women in their 30's, 40's and 50's and are noticing skin laxity because you'll need to have a fair amount of dermal thickness for your skin to respond to the treatment. They won't offer much benefit if the skin is extremely loose or saggy. In this case most doctors would recommend surgery along with the skin tightening procedure.

In most cases, for the best results, a series of treatments are needed (at approximately $500-1,000 per treatment). The results are cumulative and you are most likely to notice the full results in about 3 months. Many people are very pleased with the results, however, since there is such a variability since each person's results vary depending on the quality of his or her skin.

The duration of the results are sketchy, we couldn't get any one doctor to commit on a timeline for lasting results, however, it would appear that they can at least reset the clock back a few years so that the skin will begin aging from a new starting point. In this new age of technology newer and better devices are coming on the market every few months.

For example, **Primaeva**, which uses bipolar radiofrequency technology, will be available within the next few months in the United States. It uses needles to puncture the skin and goes deeper than current devices and will only need one session to see optimal results. **Ulthera** is another new machine out this year that uses high-frequency ultrasound to deliver energy to the deepest layers of the skin of the eyebrows and lower face to target the muscle layer typically addressed in a facelift. All of this in one treatment with no incisions!

SELPHYL - The New Non-Surgical Platelet Rich Plasma Facelift

At the most recent annual convention hosted by the American Society of Plastic Surgeons in Seattle, Washington, Dr. Joseph Gryskiewicz introduced SELPHYL, a new regeneration technology that produces an injectable serum from the patient's own blood to treat wrinkles and skin depressions. Developed by Aesthetic Factors, SELPHYL is a platelet-rich fibrin matrix (PRFM), a completely natural autologous tissue regeneration technology that has peaked the interest of plastic surgeons all over the world.

How It Works

Plastic Surgeons or dermatologists draw a small volume of blood from the patient and, through a patented process, the SELPHYL™ System separates and concentrates the patient's own blood platelets and fibrin into a matrix. The resulting serum (PRFM) is then injected into a treatment area (face or body) to stimulate cell proliferation, which promotes the increase of volume and rejuvenation of the skin through a process of guided tissue regeneration.

Dr. Gryskiewicz explained that pronounced effects occur as early as three weeks after the procedure. The effects have been shown to last beyond a year and a half in clinical studies in Japan as well as in the US at a cost of approximately $1,100 per treatment session. SELPHYL™ PRFM treats the root cause of the problem by triggering the production of new cells and collagen. The technology has received FDA 510(k) class II clearance and obtained CE Mark, which means it is approved for use in the U.S.

In a short video, Dr. Gryskiewicz showed that the entire procedure lasts less than 20 minutes in the physician's office. Compared to the current popular dermal fillers, Juvederm and

Restylane, which cost approximately $600 per 1 cc syringe, the SELPHYL™ System is highly cost effective. One blood draw will produce four 1cc syringes of serum (PRFM), possibly allowing full face rejuvenation to be performed in one session. Dr. Gryskiewicz contends that the SELPHYL™ System offers a simple, reproducible, hypoallergenic and cost-effective method of growing the patient's own tissue to fill skin depressions, wrinkles, and folds without using synthetic, plastic or animal-derived materials.

Platelet Rich Plasma therapy is currently being used in the National Football League to treat injuries, and has been used in orthopedics for 10 years without any reported complications.

The New Stem Cell Non-Surgical Facelift

It is the dawning of a new age in the world non-surgical facelifts. Stem cell technology is now being used to restore volume to the face and body. Dr. Nathan Newman, a board certified dermatologist located in Beverly Hills performs this advanced procedure.

"As we age, we lose the volume of our face and the desirable attractive and healthy proportions of the face lose their balance, causing us to look aged and tired," Dr. Newman says. "As the cheeks deflate and flatten, the height distance from the cheeks to the nose and eyes increases, causing the visual effect of the nose to protrude, making it appear larger, and causing the under eyes to appear sunken and baggy.

The Stem Cell Lift™ technique allows the cosmetic surgeon to sculpt the face and restore the pleasing and eye-catching proportions of the face without scars or the need for general anesthesia." Dr. Newman uses the ethical and non-controversial stem cells from your own body fat, known as "Autologous (self-donated) Adult Adipose Derived Mesenchymal Stem Cells". The controversial "embryonic stem cells" much debated in the media are not used.

Dr. Newman reports that the stem cells found in our fat are unique to each person. They are cells that repair and replace damaged tissues. When they are taken from one part of the body and placed in another, they become incorporated into their new environment.

Stem cells induce new collagen production, the formation of blood vessels, and the disintegration of scar tissue. They assimilate into their new home in the body, recognize their new surroundings and take on the attributes of the surrounding tissues. Stem cells are vital for the graft survival in this new environment. Once the fat is taken and is secured in the new position, the stem cells help to maintain the results for many years by ensuring adequate blood supply and by replacing older cells.

For many years doctors have been performing fat transfers, but the duration of the results were limited by the how the fat tissues was processed, lasting no longer than three years in most cases.

"In a traditional grafting procedure, the cleansing and preparation process exposed the tissues to the environment and increased the risk for contamination and infection, but more crucially it removed the stem cells as well, making them worthless," explains Dr. Newman. He says optimal long-lasting results are achieved with the STEM CELL LIFT™ which harvests the stem cells with blunt instruments that don't damage them, so they can be injected as part of the fat grafting procedure. The cell-rich fat is used to smooth and sculpt the face, with long-lasting results. The STEM CELL LIFT™ is relatively new and the cost is approximately $9,000 for the face. Results are expected to last about 9-10 years.

PART II b:

Exploring the New World of Cosmetic Surgery

§§§

Surgical Procedures

Chapter Five

The New World of Cosmetic Surgery
Surgical Procedures

Mommy Makeovers

We sat down again with Dr. Rady Rahban to learn about the popular "Mommy Makeover" that has grown to become one of the most popular procedures in the world for women of all ages. Dr. Rahban is certified by the American Board of Plastic Surgery, his specialties include breast augmentation, breast lift, rhinoplasty, tummy tuck, liposuction and facial fillers. Dr. Rahban studied and worked closely with Dr. Garth Fisher, the world renowned plastic surgeon featured on the hit ABC television show *Extreme Makeover* and had recently opened a new office in Beverly Hills.

SimplyAgeless411: We have heard so much about "Mommy Makeovers" and since they are so popular with women of all ages, can you tell us about the procedure?

Dr. RR: There is no doubt that becoming a mother is one of the most wonderful experiences a women can have. A new baby fills one's life with happiness and joy, but often leaves new mommies feeling self-conscious about the changes her body encountered during pregnancy. Despite rigorous diet and exercise routines, many mothers are unable to regain their pre-pregnancy body, leaving them frustrated and discouraged. Most women want to address the drooping breasts, loss of breast volume, stubborn pregnancy fat that won't seem to go away and of course, stretch marks.

Luckily, with the many advances in plastic surgery today, reversing the wear-and-tear on a woman's body after pregnancy and childbirth is becoming more and more common, with amazing results. The so-called "Mommy Makeover" typically includes a breast lift and/or augmentation, a tummy tuck and liposuction to safely return the body back to its pre-baby shape, perhaps even create a new and improved appearance. Your doctor can walk you through which procedures will help you reach realistic goals.

A brief description of the common procedures may allow you to determine if perhaps you are a candidate for the surgery. Breast Augmentation adds volume back into the breast through the use of a saline or silicone implant. A Breast Lift, which often is accompanied with an augmentation, not only addresses the volume loss, but recreates an attractive shape to the breast and nipple. A Tummy Tuck flattens the abdomen by removing excess skin, fat and stretch marks, as well as tightening the muscles that have stretched out considerably while carrying the baby. Finally, liposuction will remove the fat associated with "baby weight" and get rid of "love handles", the "muffin top" and "saddle bags."

Before undergoing a **"Mommy Makeover,"** it's important to that you are healthy enough post-delivery to have the surgeries and you should consider how the post-surgery recovery will affect you and your family. A Mommy Makeover isn't just for recent moms, either. Some women wait years after giving birth before considering corrective surgery. For example, if your children require constant attention (lifting/holding, etc.), you might want to consider waiting until they are a bit older. The Mommy Makeover is a wonderful option for women who have lost self-esteem from the adverse after-effects of pregnancy. Both new and veteran mommies regain their youthful appearance!

SimplyAgeless411:   Thank you so much for your time today, Dr. Rahban, this has undoubtedly provided our readers with wonderful insight into this popular procedure, and given mommies out there new hope!

Trends, Traps & Truths Behind Plastic Surgery

We think it's important to our readers to explore the business side of plastic surgery, so we sought out the counsel of a top plastic surgeon to gain a better perspective of the trends, traps and truths we should all look out for. Beverly Hills surgeon Robin Yuan, MD, graduated from Harvard Medical School and trained in general surgery at UCLA and Cedars-Sinai Medical Center. He is certified by the American Board of Plastic Surgery and has served as vice-chief of Plastic Surgery at Cedars-Sinai Hospital. He specializes in plastic surgery in all areas of the face and body.

__SimplyAgeless411__: Thank you so much for your time today, Dr. Yuan. Can you tell us a little bit about the business side of plastic surgery? What is going on behind the scenes that we should know about?

Dr. RY: Hot trends in cosmetic surgery attract surgeons, patients, and the media. The latest products and procedures get a lot of hype, which is often warranted, but each patient is different. As someone who consults with many patients for shortcomings or complications of these trends, I am more interested in truth than in the trends themselves. Being right is more important than being part of the stampeding crowd following the latest trend. In my upcoming new book, *"Behind the Mask, Beneath the Glitter,"* I devote an entire chapter to hype, reminding readers of the Gartner Hype Cycle, where technological breakthroughs, or triggers, go through a period of initial inflated expectations, followed by disillusionment, then enlightenment, and finally a plateau of productivity. Some of these advances never even get to the plateau stage and end up in the waste-yard of medical history.

The push to make an impact in our profession and on our patients is driven partly by humanism and partly by ego and, more often now, by financial gain. In the constant push for innovation, the demand of finding practical solutions to everyday problems is balanced by the fear of failure.

This is the inevitable internal debate between the pros and cons, the advantages and the disadvantages, the benefits and risks of surgical, or non-surgical, interventions. We want the cure without doing harm. We want to be in the forefront of our profession so that we don't seem out of touch with the most advanced technologies and procedures. We want to be in-the-know not in-the-dark, or out of the loop. But you do run a risk for being the first on the block to offer the latest procedures, because you are also the first one who may discover its ineffectiveness, or even dangers.

The path of modern cosmetic surgery is strewn with examples of trends that turned out to be dead ends or tragic traps: liquid silicone injections for breast and facial augmentation, soybean breast implants, ox cartilage for the nose, barbed sutures for face-lifting, cardio toxic tumescent anesthesia, the initial use of ultrasonic and laser liposuction over a decade ago, to variously ineffective lotions and potions designed to "make cellulite disappear, promote sexual drive, and increase bust size." There's always something new, the "latest thing." It is only by listening to the science, and not the media, considering the data and not the hype, that a patient can become the victor and not the victim of the trends in cosmetic surgery.

Remember that cosmetic surgery should never make you desperate for the latest trend. You will always have time to assess the effectiveness of any treatment. Any treatment should be chosen for how it can benefit you as the patient.

__SimplyAgeless411:__ Wow…this is such important information for all of us to consider and incorporate into our research process when considering any kind of plastic surgery. Thank you for enlightening us and giving us another perspective on this business.

Everything You Ever Wanted To Know About Liposuction

Since we were already sitting in one of the top plastic surgeon's office in the country, we continued our conversation by asking Dr. Robin Yuan if he would give us his opinion about the dozens of liposuction procedures currently available and provide us with a better understanding about which ones work and which ones are a waste of time and money.

SimplyAgeless411: There seems to be a new method of liposuction coming on the market every few months, in your opinion, which liposuction yields the best results?

Dr. RY: The liposuction equipment market is flooded with a host of new devices that use various forms of energy to assist in fat contouring. Ultrasound-assisted, power-assisted, water jet-assisted, laser-assisted, and radio frequency-assisted technologies all have their proponents. They all claim to produce some combination of a gentler, faster, easier, more precise, and less painful procedure. The question is whether any of these machines are truly beneficial or, more importantly, even necessary.

There is no argument that each of these technologies is effective in removing fat. Yet so is traditional liposuction with machine vacuum. Advances in technology beg the question, what is important, the tool or the craftsman, the instrument or the musician? Even those using these devices confess that technology is only as good as the surgeon using it. Having a Ferrari isn't necessary to go to the grocery store. Owning a Testarossa doesn't make you a better driver.

The problem with these technologies is that all of them effectively remove fat cells, but none of them can prevent one of the most common complications: over-suctioning, which can leave "dents" in the skin. It is better to under-suction than over-suction, since it is easier to go back for a touch-up than to try to fat graft a depression. To me, it seems unnecessary to use such high-powered devices for most patents. The majority of good candidates who have localized fat deposits and good elastic skin will fare better with traditional machine vacuum liposuction.

Liposuction is the holy grail of skin tightening. Some other machines claim to do so by generating a thermal injury under the skin to stimulate collagen formation. That will tighten the skin about 30 percent the effectiveness of traditional liposuction, and of the results, only 50 percent will be permanent. Many of the new-fangled machines out there haven't been around long enough to have a history of satisfying results. It'll take some time, so both we in the medical community and our patients will need to wait it out.

For the last decade or more, I have been predominantly using a technique called syringe liposuction. It is so simple, and seemingly crude, as to be almost laughable in today's high-tech world of "new and improved" machines. They key to its success is to use it on a patient that has a healthy, stable lifestyle, someone who takes care of themselves and doesn't use plastic surgery as a quick fix for irresponsible or sedentary behavior. Many of the patients I see who've had complications results from liposuction by another physician weren't ideal candidates living healthy lifestyles, so it was the patient, not the procedure that compromised their results.

The advantage of the syringe method is that it allows me to adjust the amount of negative pressure with each round of suctioning, so we have more control and avoid the over suctioning I mentioned earlier. More importantly, the syringe allows the control of a very exact amount of fat to be removed *before* it is actually removed. With the syringe set to 5 ccs. a precise amount of fat equivalent to 5 ccs. can be removed. Once the 5ccs. is in the syringe, suctioning is complete. If I want 17 ccs. I can suction 17ccs. If I target 58ccs., I can suction exactly 58 ccs. - no more, no less. It's precise.

With other methods, you don't know what or how much fat has been removed or destroyed until after the fact. For larger volumes of fat removal, I use a combination of machine vacuum and syringe. It's not very sexy, but it is very precise, and patients are happy with the results. My main point on this topic would be: Do not be mislead by marketing. Newer is not always better.

The Bootylicious "Butt Lift"

Living in a city like Los Angeles, we are constantly surrounded by beautiful people. At the coffee shop, the clothing boutique, clubs and restaurants, and we can't help noticing that people spend a lot of time and money on their derrieres. There are some

"Bootylicious Booties" walking around L.A. ...and we're not talking about women! Well, okay, we'll include the women.

We returned to Dr. Ryan Stanton's office to find out what procedures are popular to achieve those results that the gym cannot. Dr. Stanton is a fully credentialed board certified plastic and reconstructive surgeon who approaches cosmetic surgery by using plastic surgery on the outside and anti-aging nutrition/medicine on the inside to achieve lasting results. He told us that "buttock augmentation" and "butt lifts" are growing in popularity. Dr. Stanton has been featured in national and international media including *Discovery Channel, Women's Entertainment Network, CBS, Fox, KTLA News and Fitness.*

SimplyAgeless411: Good morning, Dr. Stanton, and thank you for meeting with us today. Tell us a little more about surgical enhancements for both men and women to achieve a great derriere?

Dr. RS: Buttock Augmentation is a solution for those who want to enhance the appearance, size and definition of the gluteal muscles in the buttocks. It adds more curvature to help sculpt the behind they desire.

SimplyAgeless411: What makes a good candidate?

Dr. RS: Simply put, any male or female who feels or perceives their buttock size, shape, or proportions are not adequate would benefit from the surgery. Many of the problems are associated with genetics or development factors, fluctuations in weight (especially weight loss), changes from pregnancy or aging, or trauma. Most of the patients I've seen have tried exercise and diet and seen some marginal results, but aren't quiet getting the look they want. That's where surgery can help.

Buttock Augmentation can be accomplished in two ways: "Autologous" (self-donated) Fat Grafting, in which your own fat is harvested, by way of liposuction, from areas of excess and then re-injected into the buttocks to mold and shape to the desired effect. Although this method works for some patients, most are not good candidates, because much of the fat dissolves over the first year after surgery, and the patients seeking to have better behinds often don't have the donor fat necessary to produce a significant, long-lasting result. Additionally, fat grafting is very labor intensive and therefore relatively expensive.

Buttock Implants (a.k.a. gluteal implants) may be a better solution for these patients. A very soft semi-solid silicone implant -- the kind that cannot rupture and leak – is placed under or within the buttock muscles through an approximately two-and-a-half inch mid-line incision overlying the tailbone. Implants come in various shapes and size but most commonly either a round (circular-domed) or ovoid (tear-drop) shape is used.

The surgery takes between and hour and a half to two hours. Typically the resulting scar is well concealed between the upper buttock cheeks. Recovery after surgery varies, but most patients can return to work after about two weeks, start exercising after four weeks, and may have unrestricted activity by six weeks. The advantages over fat grafting are that implants provide a reliable, reproducible, and relatively predictable permanent result for about only two-thirds of the cost of the fat grafting procedure.

In either case, buttock augmentation is usually done on an outpatient basis under general anesthesia. Most patients go home after a short (hour long) recovery at the surgery center. Much unlike breast augmentation with implants, buttock augmentation with implants is performed by a limited number of skilled plastic surgeons. It is crucial to have the implants placed within or under the gluteus maximus muscle.

If the implant is placed on top of the muscle it is guaranteed to migrate, usually south, and create an unappealing look. When choosing a plastic surgeon to perform this operation, make sure he/she does at least four to five buttock implants per month, because the anatomy and surgical dissection of this area is unfamiliar to many plastic surgeons.

SimplyAgeless411:   While we're here, may we ask you about a type of "Lip Enhancement" procedure that has become very popular with many women?

Dr. RS: Of course, I am happy to answer all of your questions. We do a lot of these types of procedures in my practice.

The 'Other' Lip Enhancement

SimplyAgeless411: We understand that many women have vaginal problems or defects as a result of genetics or developmental issues and others as a result of pregnancy. There are new procedures to address these issues. Can you tell us a little bit about them?

Dr. R.S: Labiaplasty and Vaginoplasty are among the fastest growing and accepted cosmetic procedures for women. It involves the surgical modification (most frequently reduction) of either the *labia minora* (inner lips) or *labia majora* (outer lips) to achieve a more proportional and/or comfortable anatomic size. The procedure is done on an outpatient basis and typically requires only light sedation or twilight sleep anesthesia.

Recovery is relatively quick, with most everyone back on their feet the next day and resuming most activities in about a week.

Sexual intercourse may commence after four weeks following labiaplasty and six weeks following vaginoplasty. Even relative to many other plastic and cosmetic surgeries, *labiaplasty* and *vaginoplasty* patients have a high satisfaction rate and an improved self-esteem after surgery.

Labiaplasty is in a category of vaginal plastic surgeries known as *female genital cosmetic surgery* (FGCS). FGCS also includes:

1. *Hoodectomy*, whereby excessive tissue covering the clitoris is reduced to provide better clitoral stimulation and improved sexual arousal.
2. *Vaginal Rejuvenation*, in which the vaginal vault is tightened and supported to provide better accommodation and thus heightened sensation during sex.

If you are a good candidate, and if necessary, *labiaplasty, vaginoplasty, hoodectomy, vaginal rejuvenation and/or vaginal reconstruction* can often be performed at the same time for convenience and to avoid multiple recovery periods.

SimplyAgeless411: What makes a good candidate for *labiaplasty* and/or *vaginoplasty*?

Dr. RS: Women with the following concerns:

Aesthetic Concerns:

- Excessive length, thickness, bulk, redundancy, and/or dark pigmentation

- Asymmetry with one side significantly larger than the other

- Deflation and/or loose skin of the labia majora (outer lips)

Functional Concerns:

- Discomfort and/or displeasure during sex

- Discomfort wearing certain clothing or when exercising or even sitting

__SimplyAgeless411__: Thank you so much for your time today, Dr. Stanton. While many women are concerned about these issues, some are uncomfortable asking questions about what's available to them. This is valuable information that I know our readers will appreciate.

The Changing Face of Cosmetic Surgery: Demographics & Attitudes

According to a recent study by the *American Society of Plastic Surgery*, even in the toughest economic times, people are still seeking out both surgical and non-surgical procedures. Patients from all walks of life are embracing what technologies are now available that we didn't have even a few years ago. It's a testament to the mainstream acceptance of cosmetic surgery. We wall want to be healthy, and to look as good on the outside as we feel on the inside.

We once again sought out the expertise of Newport Beach, California, plastic surgeon Edward Domanskis, to get his thoughts on the changing perceptions and mainstream appeal of cosmetic surgery. Certified by the American Board of Plastic Surgery, Dr. Domanskis is President and Founder of the American Society of Bariatric Plastic Surgeons and a member of the American Society of Plastic Surgery and the American Society of Aesthetic Plastic Surgery. He is listed among *America's Top Physicians and America's Best Doctors,* and appears regularly on numerous television programs, including *The Today Show, Good Morning America, 48HRS, Inside Edition,* and *EXTRA*

SimplyAgeless411: Good morning Dr. Domanskis. We have seen some of the procedures you have performed on television, and are thrilled to have you speak to us today! Why do you think more and more people are turning to plastic surgery?

Dr. E.D: There may be several reasons for this phenomenon, besides the reality television shows. Although beauty is an age-old quest, present culture has placed an extreme emphasis on appearance. You only need to glance through any magazine or watch any movie. The stigma of cosmetic surgery is gone. The majority of patients talk freely about their surgery or wanting and anticipating it! It's not a taboo subject. To look your best by whatever means possible has not only become acceptable, but actually desirable. Your neighbor, co-worker, even the teen next door is having liposuction, breast enlargement and facial rejuvenation, or so-called "extreme makeovers." They likely are financing their cosmetic surgery or paying with their credit cards because they see the value it can bring to their sense of confidence and self-esteem.

SimplyAgeless411: What other kinds of demographic changes are you seeing?

Dr. ED: No longer is cosmetic surgery just for women. Increasingly, men and those with minor imperfections are having work done.

SimplyAgeless411:   What are some of the latest procedures and techniques that you are excited about?

Dr. ED: The art and field of plastic cosmetic surgery has evolved with new and more effective procedures. Let us talk about some of these exciting techniques that have allowed plastic surgeons to keep the facial "clock turned back". These not only involve long-lasting surgical solutions, but also temporary ones. One of the most common temporary solutions that is widely talked about in the media is BOTOX. Botox is a toxin that is injected to paralyze the offending muscle, reducing the appearance of fine lines and wrinkles. The most common areas that it improves are the frown lines and the "crow's feet" area around the eyes. On average, the effects last three to five months. In some instances, it can prevent necessary movements like closing of the eyelids, which is, fortunately, temporary.

Once the facial lines are established, fillers to efface them are available. They are by-products of animals, humans or synthetics like COLLAGEN, FASCIAN, Restylane, Radience, and Juvederm. The plethora of these products attests to their limited and transient effectiveness.

Textural skin changes, primarily the result of sun damage, require different solutions. Creams, lotions and potions have all been used with some limited success. Products that break down the impenetrable skin layer fair the best. Again, the list is long and includes acids in various dilutions, abrasive chemicals, scrubs, and dermabrasion.

Most of these have been replaced by the laser, which gives the surgeon a more precise and effective tool to dramatically erase unwanted lines and reverse aging and improve sun-damaged skin. The more effective lasers work by actually burning the skin. The deeper the laser penetrates, the longer and more unpleasant the recovery, but the more significant and longer lasting the results.

Scarring and pigment changes can occur. The downtime has been shortened by fractionated technology. This Fraxcel CO2 laser, as well as Thermage (radiofrequency waves which shrink the skin) is gaining in popularity, with the former for texture changes and the latter for actual collagen tightening.

SimplyAgeless411: It seems like the traditional invasive facelift is becoming obsolete. We see trends developing where "mini-lifts" are being done with very little "cutting" involved. Can you tell us a little bit about this?

Dr. ED: The most recent significant advance in facial cosmetic surgery is primarily because of the endoscope. The endoscope is a hollow, rigid tube that emits a powerful light and features a camera that projects a highly magnified image onto a video screen. The precision and accuracy this allows for means that there is less need for more invasive surgery to achieve the same result, which of course means less scarring and recovery for the patient.

The plastic surgeon inserts specialized instruments through small one-inch access incisions hidden in the hair and guides them, not by direct visualization, but, indirectly, by what he sees on the video screen. By making small cuts, the surgeon can reposition the deep soft tissues of the face. These tissues of the face are re-suspended upwards, exactly the reverse of their descent, rather than in a front to back direction as with a traditional facelift. It's important to note that this does *not* replace the traditional facelift, because no skin is removed. When excess skin is already present, forming jowls or looseness of the face and neck, then a traditional facelift is the best course of action. Advances have been made in this area also that may shorten the length of the cuts and prolong the rejuvenating effects.

My personal techniques have evolved over many years. It's been a long time since I performed an "ear-to-ear" forehead lift, what most people associate with a traditional face lift. I expect the day is coming when cutting and the resultant scarring will become a thing of the past! Plastic surgery continues to evolve and keep pace with the demands of the ever growing and aging population striving to look better and younger.

SimplyAgeless411: As always, you have provided us with a wealth of information. Thank you, Dr. Domanskis.

Action Plan

for Cosmetic Surgery

In Your 20s: This is the time that you may consider treatments such as micro-dermabrasion to refine your skin texture, and IPL lasers to even out your skin tone. In your late 20s, you may need a series of very light facial peels such as the Jessner Peel or a Pumpkin Enzyme Peel to reduce the appearance of fine lines and roughness. Some people in this age group get a small amount of Botox injected into their frown lines. This is a good preventative measure.

After two to three years of using Botox, the latest data shows that it is needed less often (every six months instead of every 3-4) because the muscles learn to relax. On rare occasions, a person in their 20s may need a brow-lift if they have very low-set brows, which is genetic. Very low brows can give a person an angry or tired look. The other popular surgeries for this age group are rhinoplasty (nose job), breast augmentation, and lipsosuction.

In Your 30s: Many people in their 30s start getting fillers to enhance their lips and to fill their nasal labial lines. On occasion they may also correct the shape of their nose with fillers instead of having a nose job. Botox is now used for forehead lines, crow's feet, and frown lines. It is also used for over active sweat glands of the face, hands or armpits. For people with adult acne, "intra-dermal Botox" seems to be miraculous: for fading acne scars and pore tightening.

"Mommy makeovers" that include breast lifts and augmentation plus a tummy tuck and liposuction are very popular for women in their 30s into their 40s. People in their 30s get brow lifts, nose jobs, chin implants, and eyelid surgeries. Liposuction and mesotherapy are used to refine body proportions. Some young men have chin implants in conjunction with neck liposculpting to achieve a more masculine well-defined jawline. Facials get more aggressive combining microdermabrasion facials in conjunction with light peels, oxygen therapy and topically applied vitamins. Laser light therapies such as the IPL, LED Light, and Radio Frequency lasers refine the skin with almost no down time.

In Your 40s: This is the decade when most people start considering more serious surgical and non-surgical cosmetic procedures. The skin is more elastic in your 40s and will heal faster with better results than in later years. The goal is to gently turn back the clock and restore the face and body's youthfulness. "Natural" and "Refreshed" are the key words to describe what most patients want. Lasers, fat transfers, fillers and Botox can often stave off the need for facial surgery or work beautifully in conjunction. Re-volumizing the face is the gold standard. The "pulled cosmetic surgery look" becomes a thing of the past.

Liposuction, mesotherapy, and liposculpture in conjunction with skin tightening lasers and radio frequency procedures such as The Titan, Thermage, Skintyte, Polaris and ReFirm help restore a body's youthfulness. Tummy tucks, arm lifts, and leg lifts are popular for people in this age group as well as breast lifts, augmentations, breast reductions and labiaplasties.

Laser resurfacing procedures such as the fractionated CO2 laser and the Cool Touch Erbium laser help rebuild lost collagen of the face, neck, chest, and hands creating a tightening effect three to four months after treatment. The fractionated lasers also gently resurface the skin, removing years of sun damage and discoloration as well as tightening the skin with less than a week of downtime.

Hyaluronic based fillers such as Juvederm, Restylane, and Perlane are now used more extensively to add volume to the lips, lift the brow, revolumize the cheeks and hollows of the face, fill out the jawline, fill in under eye circles, and much more, all while actually stimulating new collagen production in the skin! Radiesse is another popular dermal filler. It is made of calcium hydroxyapatite, which is a substance that is made from minerals that give your bones strength and texture. The minerals are formulated by grinding them into microscopic particles; these particles are then suspended in a water-based gel solution.

Sculptra, a more permanent filler, is used for total facial revolumizing for larger areas of the face. Rejuvenating the entire face with injectible fillers together with Botox, is called the "Liquid Face Lift". This is the most popular method of facial rejuvenation and can help stave off the need for surgery for many years. The most popular facial surgeries for "forty somethings" are blepharoplasties (upper and/or lower eye lid surgery) browlifts, and mini-face lifts that tighten the jawline and lower face.

In Your 50s and Beyond: This is the time when most people opt for more invasive cosmetic procedures. Keep in mind that for many people no amount of fillers, Botox or laser/chemical resurfacing can repair the underlying issue of muscle laxity and sagging skin. Therefore cosmetic surgery procedures such as the full facelift, necklift, upper and lower eyelid surgery, mid-face lift to reposition the cheek pads that have dropped, a brow lift, are in high demand. These procedures in conjunction with all other procedures will maintain your appearance to a youthful level throughout your life. The most popular cosmetic surgery procedures for people in their 50s and beyond are:

- Medical skin care

- Laser hair removal
- Laser Light based treatments
- Microdermabrasion
- Botox
- Chemical peels
- Injectible fillers
- Botox
- Laser skin resurfacing
- Tummy tucks
- Breast augmentation/lifts/reductions
- Browlifts
- Eyelid surgeries
- Facelifts
- Mid-face lifts
- Liposuction
- Necklifts
- Nose reshaping

Maintaining good health habits, doing regular exercise (including weight bearing exercises), having monthly facials, using facial fillers and Botox, keeping your hormones and thyroid levels strong and balanced plus having the right cosmetic surgery procedures will keep you looking fresh and vibrant. It is unrealistic to believe that one procedure alone will get you to your goals of a youthful appearance. While we will never look twenty forever, we can look refreshed, rested and beautiful/handsome our entire lives. More and more *"No Age is The New Age."*

PART III

The New World of Cosmetic Dentistry

Chapter Six

Creating a Dazzling Smile
The New Age of Cosmetic Dentistry

As we grow older, the subtle changes to the structures of our faces begin gradually and then pick up speed after about 40. Our chins move back, our cheeks hollow and wrinkles appear. Additionally, as we age our jaws recede and our faces shorten. These changes can be partially reversed by remolding teeth, which are part of the scaffolding of the face, to restore your face to its original structure.

Several dentists we interviewed told us that when the teeth are in the right position, it fills out the volume of the face. Additionally, when you see more teeth, it is a brighter and more refreshed and youthful appearance. Procedures vary widely, from changing a few teeth to a total remake of a person's bite. Most procedures involve adding length or bulk because teeth tend to shorten from normal use with and, in some patients, years of night grinding. By slightly thickening side teeth for example, dentists can create a wider area over the lip, smoothing wrinkles.

Typically, it involves placing porcelain veneers over existing teeth; however, some dentists use a white-colored bonding material that can be added to teeth to re-sculpt their shape. Lengthening front teeth is a key component of many procedures. According to a 1978 study by scientists at the University of California School of Dentistry, people under 29 show an average of 3.37 millimeters of their upper teeth with lips gently parted in a resting position, compared with less than half a millimeter when they reach their 50s.

There are so many new advancements in cosmetic dentistry today. We needed the expert opinions of two of the top dentists in Los Angeles. Dr. Kourosh Maddahi graduated top in his class at UCLA, then received his dental doctorate from USC. He is well known for his skill and artistry in cosmetic and restorative work.

SimplyAgeless411:   Good morning, Dr. Maddahi. We know you have a busy schedule so we'll get right to the point. What are the most important ways a person's teeth can look more youthful and better?

Dr. M: There are three main aspects that affect the youthfulness of a smile: The harmony of the teeth, the color of the teeth and the shape of the teeth.

SimplyAgeless411: What is the first thing that you evaluate when you meet a new patient?

Dr. M: I look at the harmony of the teeth and then of the face. No tooth should be longer or shorter than the others, since that attracts unwanted attention to the teeth and distracts from the overall smile. Here are other elements of a smile that I evaluate:

- Lip support: if the upper and lower lips are in proper proportion and in the right place.
- The complexion of the skin: the lighter the complexion, the lighter the teeth. If a patient doesn't have a lot of natural contrast, such as in dark skin tone, then the color of the teeth and the complexion come into play. Otherwise they can look fake and unnatural.
- Whether a patient uses the following: green tea, coffee, or smokes. If they do, when choosing the color of the veneers, I go a shade to two lighter for the color of their teeth, to compensate for any staining that will occur.
- How much teeth structure or gums/ gum line shows. Too much gums showing detracts from the beauty of the smile and the person.

- Relationship of the upper teeth to the lower teeth. Overbites and underbites create challenges as to the degree of improvement possible.

- If they have red hair, real or fake: I need to go one-two shades lighter on their teeth or grayness is reflected because of the red hair.

- If the shape of the upper teeth follows the curvature of the lower lip when they smile. That's how I know if someone's teeth are too long. I must see if there is proper curvature.

- The actual arch of the upper and lower teeth. You should have a nice arch form from the back to the front to form a nice smile. This determines the thickness of the veneers/crowns. If you see a black hole when people smile at the back of the teeth, then I would need to compensate by making the outer side of their molars thicker to broaden the appearance of their arch.

SimplyAgeless411: What is the most important talent a cosmetic dentist must have?

Dr. M: A great cosmetic dentist must be able to see the end result when he examines someone's mouth. That's what separates good from great...seeing the end result even before you begin any work.

Then I work backwards from the end result I envision to the existing smile. Otherwise you are exploring, then things can come up that you don't expect, rather than pre-planning so there are no surprises. Even surprises of additional decay or fractures or unexpected problems are okay because they will be reworked and covered. The main thing is how you will cover the teeth to achieve the end result. I see the end result first in my head first, and then nothing can interfere with reaching the right goal for my patient.

SimplyAgeless411:   What is your goal for your patients' teeth?

Dr. M: My goal is perfect color, perfect shape, perfect length, and perfect arch form.

SimplyAgeless411:   You obviously have a good artistic sense. Did you learn any of this in dental school?

Dr. M: Thank you, but no, I did not learn anything about artistic style in dental school. Dental school only teaches function, not aesthetics. This is something that in my opinion cannot be taught.

SimplyAgeless411:   I know that you pride yourself in being a great listener. Why do you feel that this is so crucial to your overall success and patient satisfaction?

Dr. M: I spend a lot of time listening to what the patient needs and wants. The only thing a patient doesn't know is how white their teeth can be without looking fake. They can understand shape, but not how the color will look. Patients know the look they want. I listen intently to find out their expectations so I can meet them. I also show the patients samples of teeth colors, computer images, photographs of their improved smile and wax-ups (scale models of the completed smile). This is all done to communicate more effectively, so there are no surprises…well, perhaps some very positive ones!

SimplyAgeless411: What is the reason restored teeth look fake?

Dr. M: The main reason teeth look fake is because either they are too long or too thick. Not because they are too white. In the past ten years, the white that we used to think was good has been replaced with a much whiter white. This has been driven by the entertainment industry. These newer shades of white did not exist ten years ago. Studios are demanding good teeth now on their actors. This is a relatively new thing that started about five to seven years ago.

SimplyAgeless411: Do most people ask you to just give them a white smile?

Dr. M: Up until about 5 years ago, patients were satisfied with whiter teeth. Now patients know the limitations of whitening. Today my patients ask for "that Hollywood smile". They are more aware of what is possible.

SimplyAgeless411:   What are the things that a patient should look for when choosing a cosmetic dentist?

Dr. M: The dentist should be able to listen to the patient and find out exactly what they are looking for... and is willing to educate the patient as to what's achievable. So much of cosmetic dentistry is personal preference. The dentist should be able to duplicate what the patient wants if it is at all possible. The main points are:

- The doctor should be a cosmetic dentistry specialist with many years of experience, and with a practice that focuses exclusively on cosmetic dentistry.
- The dentist should have worked on many cases similar to yours... you don't want to be the guinea pig.
- They should be able to provide at least three references of patients.
- The cleanliness of the office, the staff, if you feel comfortable with them and if they seem trustworthy.

- Education: there is no actual degree in cosmetic dentistry, so it's basically the expertise and experience of that doctor. Ask them about their education.

- The artistic sense of the doctor. Does it match your artistic sense? Look at before and after photos of past patients.

- The technology of the office: Do they have good before/after pictures? Is the office computerized? Do they have lasers and machines: With computers dentists can take images instead of impressions and the tooth is made on the spot with the computer and a milling machine. Do they offer this technology?

- With lasers: fillings of cavities can be done with laser light, as can gum lifts. Lasers of the future will be able to clean teeth with different spectrums of light and remove tartar and plaque (all up for FDA approval). Bacteria will be killed easily with laser light. Is your dentist already talking about this technology?

- Do they have a digital bite recorder for better accuracy?

- Do they offer digital x-rays?

- Do they use a digital cat scan for taking an image of the jaw to see quality of the bone, to find infections in the sinus, length and integrity of the bone for implants, intra-oral picture of the teeth, bite and jawbones?

- Can they offer 3D imaging to reconstruct the person's jaw and face: preplanned before the patient arrives for surgery? This saves months of time and makes for superior comfort and accuracy.

- The caliber of the staff. Does the staff knows how to use the technology in the office and are they are well trained doing so?

SimplyAgeless411: Wow...that is a great comprehensive list! Please tell us more about the new breakthroughs in the world of cosmetic dentistry:

Dr. M:.

1. Whitening is now being done mostly with laser light. Trays are for 20 min touch ups at home, but not used in the dentist's office anymore. Two weeks of the trays have been replaced by 1-2 hours of laser light tooth whitening in the office.

2. Re-contouring of the teeth for minimal chips and unevenness is more common now.

3. Porcelain veneers and crowns are used more than tooth bonding. Bonding stains 10 times more than porcelain and chips and breaks.

4. Metal fillings are a thing of the past. They have been replaced with porcelain and smaller fillings with tooth-colored bondings.

5. Gum line restoration is something that wasn't done a few years ago, but is a common practice now.

6. Replacement of missing teeth with dental implants. This rejuvenates the face and makes it fuller again. Dentures and missing teeth both make the face sink in. With implants a person can have normal facial structure.

7. Straightening some degree of crooked teeth without braces. This is for minimal correction that doesn't change the bit or function of the teeth.

8. We also provide referral for lip rejuvenation/fillers to complete and balance the total smile.

SimplyAgeless411: Is there anything that can't be fixed?

Dr. M: *Everything can be fixed.* Even bone grafting can be done if necessary, by taking bone from the hip or another area of the body. The good news is that there is no longer any reason, apart from the expense, why a person can't have a beautiful healthy smile.

SimplyAgeless411: How would a patient know how their smile would look after having cosmetic dentistry?

Dr. M: They can see cosmetic images and wax up models that show them how their smile can look with properly done cosmetic dentistry.

SimplyAgeless411: How long does full mouth restoration take?

Dr. M: The average time for full mouth reconstruction is two weeks, two visits and a follow-up bite adjustment.

SimplyAgeless411: Is cosmetic dentistry very painful?

Dr. M: There is little to no discomfort compared to years ago. Patients are usually delightfully surprised.

SimplyAgeless411: Do you ever feel like you have enough new equipment or technology in your practice?

Dr. M: No, never. I always want to be the first to offer the newest and the best technological advances for my patients to increase their comfort, results and speed of treatment.

SimplyAgeless411: It sounds like the future of cosmetic dentistry is already here!

Dr. M: It is in my office and continues to get better every year.

SimplyAgeless411: Now that is exciting!

Encouraged by Dr. Maddahi's comments, we next met with Dr. Dean Carlston. A graduate of Baylor Dental School, Dr. Carlston's practice features cosmetic dentistry (including Invisalign & Lumineers) and biomimetic dentistry, which is a new technology that focuses on tooth conservancy. It treats weak, fractured, and decayed teeth in a way that keeps them strong, and protects them from harmful bacteria. This innovation has practically eliminated the need to grind teeth down for crowns and destructive root canal treatment. Dr. Carlston is also an arch development specialist for young children. His practice participates in a program where his patients can "bank" their own stem cells from extracted teeth, to harvest later if needed for other procedures as they get older.

SimplyAgeless411: Dr. Carlston, tell us about the latest developments in cosmetic dentistry from your perspective, and what you are able to provide to your patients?

Dr. D.C.: There are some exciting new developments in the world of both anti-aging and cosmetic dentistry. For example, I had a patient come in with a tooth that had turned dark from a previous root canal. Although the tooth really needed a more substantial restoration, she was out the door in 30 minutes with a matching tooth in her smile. She was delighted. That's something we wouldn't have been able to offer a few years ago.

SimplyAgeless411: Wow…how did you do that?

Dr. D.C.: We accomplished this with the brand new **Paint-On Whitener** created by DenMat, which is the same company that brought us Lumineers. The **Paint-On Whitener** is applied much like fingernail polish, and gives our patients an immediate whiter and more uniform smile. It comes in different shades, can be applied in one visit with no shots and lasts for about six months before it needs a touching up. **Paint-On Whitener** is perfect for those wanting a quick fix for a special occasion or for those who are unable to bleach their teeth because of sensitivity. They are also an alternative to the standard, more expensive veneers. **Paint-On Whitener** is ideal for a single tooth, several teeth, or an entire smile!

SimplyAgeless411: Can you give us more specifics on how it works?

Dr. D.C.: It's comprised of 80 percent glass and 20 percent resin, and is applied only to the front of the tooth for cosmetic purposes. It should only be done by a qualified dentist, but there are no side effects and it causes no harm to the health of the tooth. It's also reversible and can easily be ground away without damaging the tooth. Regular veneers done by a high-end quality provider would cost anywhere from $1,000 to $2,000 each. Some more "exclusive" providers charge much more, but the quality isn't any better if they are applied by a good dentist with experience in working with them. By contrast, the **Paint-On Whitener** costs on average $300 per tooth. This means a patient can pay $1,800 for the 6 front teeth, where they would spend $6,000 to $12,000, and above, for porcelain.

SimplyAgeless411: These quick fixes are amazing and can really save the day for special occasions! Out here in Los Angeles, we hear about all kinds of interesting cosmetic tricks. Can you tell us about the new "Snap-On Smiles?"

Dr. D.C.: Yes, of course. A confident and beautiful smile is just a snap away…no shots, no drilling, no adhesives and you can even eat with it.

SimplyAgeless411: Fascinating…do tell us more!

Dr. D.C.: The **Snap-On Smile** is a thin, flexible, specialized resin material fabricated to snap over your actual teeth and can be removed like any dental appliance. The material can be made as thin as .5mm without compromising strength. You can choose from 23 color shades and 18 smile designs. It's great for people who are looking for that celebrity smile but don't have the red carpet budget.

The Snap-On-Smile is the affordable cosmetic alternative to permanent dental work - priced at a fraction of the cost of a full set of porcelain veneers or crowns. It provides a viable restorative option for all patients - particularly those who are dental phobic, financially challenged, or medically compromised. I often use these appliances to give my patients a preview of how they will look after extensive full mouth rehabilitation, where we completely change their smile through a combination of orthodontic and cosmetic procedures. For example, a gentleman was getting married and did not want to start his orthodontic treatment prior to the marriage, so we created the snap-on smile to mask his natural teeth, which were misaligned and discolored. The appliance gave him the confidence to meet all of the new in-laws and smile for the wedding photos. He will start his extensive rehabilitation treatment after he settles in with his new bride!

SimplyAgeless411:   How much does a Snap-On Smile cost?

Dr. D.C.:   Of course, the cost varies from city to city, but we charge $1,500 for a complete arch, which is a complete set of upper or lower teeth. They really don't make them with fewer teeth, because those teeth covered become longer, wider and thicker; and it looks strange not to fill out the entire arch. Most people elect the Snap-On Smile as a temporary solution while they save up for the more permanent reconstruction.

These appliances are especially great for the patient considering Lumineers, which are thin veneers that are bonded to the teeth with no or very little natural tooth reduction. Because Lumineers also give you a broader, fuller smile, the patient is able to get a preview of the final look with a snap-on smile and feel comfortable about their decision. It's a way of "test-driving" your smile.

SimplyAgeless411: These new advancements in cosmetic dentistry are really incredible. Just one more thing before we go: can you give us some of your top tips for taking care of our teeth and keeping them their whitest without undergoing any cosmetic dentistry?

Dr. D.C.: The top response to a poll we did asking people what they thought made a smile unattractive was "yellow, discolored or stained teeth". Understand that coffee, tea, dark sodas, red wine, blueberries, and tobacco all stain the teeth; so, if and when you consume these substances, use a straw with the liquids to allow them to bypass the teeth.

To get rid of stains, you can brush your teeth with a mixture of baking soda and 3 percent hydrogen peroxide (the type used in cuts and on blemishes). I also encourage patients to chew sugarless gum containing Xylitol, a sweetener extracted from the bark of the birch tree. This sweetener inhibits bacterial growth and reduces the ability of plaque to cling to the tooth surface. Xylitol makes the teeth feel like they are slick and smooth

Chewing gum sweetened with Xylitol also causes increased salivary flow. The saliva has a slightly alkaline chemistry that neutralizes the acids that wreak such havoc on the teeth. I purchase Spry Xylitol gum from VP Discounts, 100 pieces per container for around $8.00. I keep a container in my car and office, and chew a piece after each snack throughout the day.

Chewing raw crunchy vegetables is also very helpful since the fiber "brushes and cleans the teeth." The alkalines in raw vegetables help neutralize the acids in the mouth, not to mention the fact that vegetables are good for you! I can guarantee that if you eat several servings of raw vegetables throughout the day your hygienist will tell you have less tartar build up!

If you want a brighter, more even smile, talk to your dentist about straightening them first with braceless Invisalign trays, then, either whitening them or covering them with porcelain veneers, Lumineers, or paint-on composite material.

SimplyAgeless411:   One of the reasons we wanted to visit with you today was to learn more about Biomimetic Dentistry...a relatively new field of anti-aging or holistic dentistry. We understand that you are one of a handful of doctors in the United States practicing Biomimetic Dentistry. Please tell us all about it.

Dr. D.C.:   Biomimetic Dentistry means that the dentist, while restoring a diseased tooth, attempts to mimic the biological makeup of the natural tooth. We restore infected teeth while preserving as much natural tooth structure as possible. As Science has advanced in developing ultra-sensitive testing machines, we have learned that even the crown, that part of the tooth we see when we smile, has a flex to it when we chew. Finely tuned instruments can tell us how much flex the enamel and dentin have, and we can then compare this data to restorative materials that have been developed through the years. With the advent of the wonderful adhesives that dentists now have at their disposal, we are able to bond composite and porcelain restorations to those parts of the tooth that have become diseased. We can do this conservatively, preserving more of the natural tooth.

Feldspathic porcelain flexes similar to enamel, (the outer shell of the crown), and composite materials flex similar to dentin, (the structure underneath the enamel). In restoring damaged teeth, Biomimetic Dentists choose the proper material and adhesive that most closely matches that part of the tooth being restored.

SimplyAgeless411: It's so nice to know that we can now look forward to a lot less drilling and a lot more preservation of our natural teeth the next time we need a crown! Thank you so much for these great tips, Dr. Carlston.

Action Plan

for Cosmetic Dentistry

In Your 20s: This is the time to take your smile seriously by forming good habits that will help your teeth last a lifetime. Keep your sugar intake to a minimum. Avoid sugary sodas. Eat raw vegetables. Be certain to get sufficient calcium and vitamin D3 on a daily basis. Rinse your mouth after meals and chew gum made with Xylitol to help reduce plaque. Floss at least once a day and brush at least two times a day with a soft toothbrush. Have your teeth cleaned twice a year. Get your teeth whitened and repair any chips, gaps or unevenness in your teeth. Consider adult orthodonture to straighten your teeth with invisible braces.

In Your 30s: As your career blossoms, your smile becomes more important than ever. White, clean, even, smooth teeth are a mark of education, status and good health. Drinking coffee, tea and red wine take their toll on the color of your teeth. Have your teeth professionally whitened with Zoom or BriteSmile. Get at-home whitening trays custom made for maintenance. Have your smile assessed by a cosmetic dentist to get a first class smile, which may include getting porcelain veneers, tooth painting, bonding, and crowns. After the age of 35, one usually sees the first onset of gum disease. Good nutrition, the right vitamins, and very good oral hygiene are essential. Proper brushing, flossing and using mouthwash on a daily basis are crucial. Mouthwash combats inflammation of the gums (bleeding gums).

In Your 40s: The focus now must be on gum maintenance. Healthy gums and bones are the main considerations. It's essential to have your teeth cleaned 3-4 times a year now instead of only twice to avoid gingivitis and receding gum lines. Bleeding gums are often a sign of hormonal changes and imbalances.

More coffee and sugar intake to combat fatigue can take a toll on your teeth. Green tea is the most staining, although the more healthy choice. Years of drinking green tea, coffee and red wine almost always changes the color of your teeth completely. Teeth whitening and veneers are used to give you a white smile once again. For tooth loss, dental implants are much more desirable now than bridges or removable apparatus because in your forties, your bones are stronger and more dense than in later years. This is the time to "repair and restore" your smile.

In Your 50s: Clenching and grinding or the teeth often takes its toll. Wear and tear on the jaw muscles can actually change and crowd the position of the lower teeth. Clenching changes the lower jar and creates movement. Due to this, many people in their 50s experience more crowding in the lower front teeth. It's imperative to get a night guard or a retainer to combat the detrimental effects of clenching and grinding or the shape of the face can actually change. The lower lip often times starts to stick out, while the upper lip tends to get thinner…all due to the teeth repositioning in an unhealthy way.

Porcelain crowns and veneers are used to move the teeth into the correct arch. The lips regain more fullness as building up the teeth gives more upper lip support. The shape of the face regains a more balanced shape. This is often referred to as a "dental face lift". Adult orthodontia is another alternative, but can take up to two to three years versus two to three visits for reconstructive cosmetic dentistry.

PART IV

A New Age in Skincare
Age-Proofing Your Skin from the
Inside Out

Chapter Seven

The Anti-Aging Guide To Skincare
What You Need to Know

There is so much new technology out there, making so many new products, discoveries and even delivery systems – lipids, peptides, serums, potions, lotions, etc., that it's hard to know who or what to believe. In this chapter, we will help you navigate your way through the new world of anti-aging skincare products.

We make several recommendations in this chapter based on the information acquired through numerous physician interviews. We do not receive compensation, advertising fees or any kind of barter agreements for mentioning these products. Our mission in this book is to provide you with bottom-line unbiased information from some of the top physicians and medical specialists in the world.

Around your late 20s and 30s, and into your 40s and 50s, the signs of skin-aging begin. You will start noticing changes in the texture of your skin and depending on the lighting, your skin may appear to be dimpling and wavy on various areas of your body. Your skin may also appear to be thin and creppy. This is primarily because of depleting collagen levels, which, up until now, we could do very little to prevent. The new advancements in skin-tightening, such as radio-frequency, lasers and infrared light technology that we discussed in Part 2 of this book go a long way to improve skin texture and keep it youthful. To have a lifetime of beautiful skin, men and women need to do five important things as part of their skin care regimen:

1. Exercise
2. Maintain a balanced diet rich in healthy oils, proteins, fruits and greens
3. Limit exposure to environmental factors such as the sun and cigarette smoke
4. Use topical skincare products such as sunscreens, exfolliants, hyaluronic acid serums, moisturizers & retinoids (a synthetic form of Vitamin A)
5. Opt for medical grade nutritional supplements. Did you know that by taking daily vitamin C and fish oil supplements you can increase the skin's elasticity by approximately 14 percent?

Two Major Categories of Anti-Aging Skincare:

<u>Category I</u>

I. Regeneration & Repair: – These skincare products attack and repair symptoms such as fine lines, sagging skin, discoloration, spots, wrinkles, laxity, etc. When you're shopping for these products you are actively looking to repair and regenerate the skin. Let's drill down and take a deeper look into skin rejuvenation products:

<u>Skin Regeneration</u>

The glow of youth is lost over the years as the outer layer of the epidermis becomes thick and opaque. Some skincare products actually do create change. For instance, they can help restore the luster of skin on the outside and create better skin health from the inside. After interviewing some of the top dermatologists in the U.S., we have developed the follow list of recommended products.

<u>Neo Strata:</u> Alpha Hydroxy acids are one example of skincare products that actually produce a direct, measurable change in skin texture. The purpose of hydroxy acid products is two-fold: 1.) To produce a smoother texture and even color and 2.) to help in acne-prone skin. NeoStrata (glycolic based) was founded and managed

by Drs. Eugene Van Scott and Ruey Yu, who are the world recognized experts in glycolic acid research.

Eminence Cranberry Pomegranate Sugar Scrub – For those who prefer to use their alpha hydroxy in a scrub. Eminence is made of sugars containing powerful antioxidants in cranberry, pomegranate, green tea, and grape seed oil to protect your body from damage as you polish away all your dead skin cells. It's ideal for all skin types to exfoliate dead skin cells, moisturize the skin, and infuse nutrition into it. Cranberry is rich in Vitamin C, which brightens and tones the skin. Raw Sugar Cane acts as a natural, exfoliating Alpha Hydroxy Acid. Pomegranate is a rich antioxidant that protects the skin from damaging free radicals.

NIA 24 – A skin strengthening repair cream that was tested at the National Cancer Institute and has been shown to reverse DNA damage. This product is very important for people with fair skin who have had sun damage – even severe damage. Some of the benefits of NIA 24 include a softening of color irregularity and a reduction in scaling, precancerous growths. It can reduce the prevalence of skin cancer at the same time is minimizes the effects of overexposure to the sun.

RevaléSkin Cream: is a relatively new product on the market, and the first to use caffeine extracted from the coffee berry as a powerful anti-oxidant. It reduces lines and fine wrinkles from moderate sun damage.

Retin-A/Renova - Vitamin-A creams fall into both the Rejuvenation and Anti-Aging categories because they repair sun-damaged and aging skin. They also help prevent precancerous lesions and skin cancer. Everyone who can tolerate them should be using one, but they are strong. Vitamin-A creams go by all sorts of names such as Renova, Retin-A, Tazorac, Tretinoin (all available by prescription only).

Retinol is a weaker form available without a prescription. But there is one Retinol product—the SkinCeuticals Retinol 1.0—which is almost as strong as the prescription form. Some men and women may experience irritation when using a vitamin-A cream, but if you have problems, first try washing with a gentle cleanser, applying a light moisturizer and then letting your skin dry for 10 to 15 minutes; then, use a pea-sized amount for your entire face.

Renova is the best for dry or over-40-skin because it has a moisturizing base. Apply these products at night because light inactivates them. You *must* use a daily sunscreen if you're using Vitamin-A creams.

Triluma is the most widely used prescription bleaching agent in the United States. It contains three prime ingredients – 4%

hydroquinone, Tretinoin, and a topical steroid. This product is excellent for color irregularities seen in photo damaged skin, especially in darker skin types.

SkinCeuticals is the leader in cosmeceutical skin care serums and advanced technology for medically driven skin care products. They actually help reverse sun damage, lighten sun spots, soften wrinkles, and more. They are perhaps most known for their C E Ferulic® serum, a revolutionary antioxidant combination that delivers advanced protection against photo-aging - neutralizing free radicals, helping build collagen, and providing unmatched antioxidant protection. Their newest revolutionary sunblock, Sheer Physical UV Defense SPF 50, is 100% natural. Made of zinc oxide (Z-COTE®) and titanium dioxide, it is enhanced by artemia salina, a plankton extract, to increase the skin's defenses and resistance to UV and heat stress.

Category II

II. Preventative Skincare – Anti-aging or preventive skin care products dominate television ads and magazine ads around the world. These are products that keep your skin looking young and vibrant and they help prevent wrinkles from becoming prominent. Some of these skincare products are designed not so much to change your face for the better, but to prevent changes from happening for the worse. Let's take a closer look at the following anti-aging skincare products and see what they do:

302 Protein Drops: This is a new topical derived from the avocado that has the unique ability to thicken both the dermis and the epidermis layers of the skin as well as help reverse thinning skin.

Replenix - uses powerful antioxidants from the polyphenols of green tea to combat aging and loss of elasticity and luster.

Retinoids /Retin-A/Renova - Vitamin-A creams fall into both the Rejuvenation and Anti-Aging categories because they repair sun-damaged and aging skin. They also help to prevent precancerous lesions and skin cancer. Vitamin-A creams go by all sorts of names like Renova, Retin-A, Tazorac, Tretinoin (all available by prescription only).

Retinol is a weaker form available without a prescription. But there is one Retinol product—the SkinCeuticals Retinol 1.0—which is almost as strong as the prescription form. Some men and women may experience irritation when using a vitamin-A cream, but if you have problems, first try washing with a gentle cleanser, applying a light moisturizer and then letting your skin dry for 10 to 15 minutes; then, use a pea-sized amount for your entire face. Renova is the best for dry or over-40-skin because it has a moisturizing base. Apply these products at night because light inactivates them. You *must* use a daily sunscreen if you're using Vitamin-A creams.

Hyaluronic Acid Topical Serum - Even though many may think that hyaluronic acid sounds like something you used during chemistry class in high school, it is actually a naturally occurring substance within the body that belongs to the class of compounds known as glycosaminoglycans (GAGs). As we grow older, the ability of the skin to produce HA (Hyaluronic Acid) decreases and the amount of functional HA begins to fall. Since HA helps to bind water, the ability of the skin to retain water also declines with age. As a result, the skin becomes drier, thinner, and less able to restore itself. The loss of skin fullness also means that the skin becomes looser. This leads to wrinkling and the older appearance of the skin. Clinically, this can be referred to as the "plum to prune, grape to raisin phenomenon."

Hyaluronic Acid (HA) will nourish, rejuvenate and restore your skin's youthful glow. HA is the body's own super moisturizer, capable of holding up to 1000 times its own weight in water. In the skin, HA's hydrating properties provide elasticity to help prevent wrinkles. Young skin is smooth and elastic and contains a large amount of HA that helps the skin look healthy.

Topical HA can help by increasing endogenous HA in the

dermis and by attracting a water layer on top of the skin surface to protect against water loss. Topically applied, HA can offset the decreased production of HA that occurs with age. It hydrates and rejuvenates the skin and improves the tone and appearance by enhancing the skin's ability to retain moisture. Applying a special HA serum that has a light, non-oily texture, can soothe skin, smooth fine lines and reduce the appearance of wrinkles.

Note**At the time of the writing of this book, it is our understanding that Medicis Corporation's **Restylane Hyaluronic Acid** topical cream will be available in the fall of 2010. However, you can currently purchase Hyaluronic Acid topical serum through Vitamin Research Products at www.VRP.com

Moisturizers

Moisturizers are an all-important part of the ongoing daily anti-aging regimen, particularly if you have dry skin. Moisturizers will help to prevent fine lines and improve the appearance of your skin. We've all had the experience of being dry, applying a moisturizer, and having our skin look instantly better.

Here are some tips on how to get the most out of your moisturizer:

- In general, if you have oily skin, use a gel moisturizer that will hydrate your skin without adding more oil.

- If you have normal skin, use a lotion or light cream.

- If you are very dry, use a heavy cream that takes a minute or two to absorb into your skin. Apply it more frequently than once or twice a day.

- *Everyone* should use a moisturizer around their eye area and on their necks, because we all have very few oil glands in those areas.

- If you're oily through the T-zone area, just use your moisturizer on your eye area, your cheeks, and your neck.

Each of the basic types of skin is both a blessing and a curse. If you have oily skin, you have your own natural moisturizer and less tendency toward wrinkles. But you'll have more of a tendency toward acne and enlarged pores.

If you have dry skin, you'll have a greater tendency toward wrinkles but much less tendency toward acne and large pores. There's something positive about each skin type.

Here are a list of moisturizers that are recommended by some of the top dermatologists that we interviewed for this book:

- MD Forte Hydrating moisturizing cream
- NeoStrata Ultra Smoothing Cream
- DDF Ultra Light Moisturizing Dew
- Cellex-C Sea Silk Oil Free Moisturizer

- Cetaphil Moisturizing Lotion—for normal, sensitive skin (available at your drugstore)

- Cetaphil Moisturizing Cream—for dry, sensitive skin (available at your drugstore)

- EstéeLauder Clear Difference Advanced Oil-Control Hydrator—for oily and blemish-prone skin (a bit more expensive; available at department stores)

- Neutrogena Healthy Skin Lotion—for normal to dry skin (available at your drugstore)

- Olay Total Restoration Lotion—for normal to dry skin (available at your drugstore)

- Neova – A copper peptide: Since 1999, copper peptide creams have been considered by many top dermatologists as one of the most effective wrinkle prevention creams available.

Cleansers

Since cleansers are only on your face for about 15 seconds twice a day there are few, if any, therapeutic effects on the skin. If you have normal to dry skin, a cleanser or gelee that doesn't dry out or strip oil off your skin works the best. Some of these products can be a little harsh so watch closely for any signs of irritation. If you have very oily skin, a cleanser that is formulated specifically for acne is the best alternative.

Here is a list of cleansers that are recommended by top dermatologists:

- Custom Dermaceuticals for Very Sensitive Skin - This product is free of most allergens in skin care products, including parabens, preservatives, and lanolin. It is gentle and mild for sensitive skin.
- MD Forte Hydrating Cleanser For Dry Skin With No Acne
- Topix Citrix Antioxidant Cleanser For Dry Skin With Acne
- MD Forte Facial Cleanser For Oily Skin With Moderate Acne
- Cetaphil Gentle Skin Cleanser—for dry or sensitive skin (available at your drugstore)
- Lancôme Galatée Confort Comforting Milky Creme Cleanser—for dry skin (available at department stores)
- Cetaphil Daily Facial Cleanser for Normal to Oily Skin— for normal to oily skin (available at your drugstore)
- Neutrogena Oil-Free Acne Wash Foam Cleanser—for oily or acne-prone skin (available at your drugstore.

Sunscreens…A Hot Topic!

It's hard to resist the warm, inviting sunshine at the beach, golf course or tennis court during the summer months when the temptation of get a "healthy-looking tan" is strong. It's just important to be aware of your exposure during the winter months too!

We asked **Dr. Norman Leaf**, a board certified plastic surgeon in Beverly Hills and a clinical and Associate Clinical Professor of Plastic Surgery at UCLA, to give us an **in-depth look into the world of over-the-counter sunscreens** and tell us what works and what doesn't. He also gives us the *411* on an exciting new wonder drug called *Dimercine* currently in FDA trials that helps reverse sun damage. Find out how to enjoy the dog days of summer without them coming back to bite you in the end.

SimplyAgeless411: Good morning, Dr. Leaf and thank you for your insight into the world of sunscreens and the new technologies on the horizon. Please tell us what we can do to protect our skin from the sun.

Dr. N.L.: We all know now that the *effects of solar radiation on the skin are permanent and progressive.* With the depletion of the protective ozone layer, there is even more reason to be aware of the need to shield yourself from the harmful rays of the sun. Danger much more lethal than mere premature aging is lurking, including basal cell and squamous cell skin cancers, and of particular concern, the potentially fatal *malignant melanoma. We have three clear choices:*

· **Do *as doctors say*, and religiously avoid unprotected sun exposure, or**

· **Do *whatever you want* and pay the inevitable consequences later, or**

· **Do *as doctors do (like me)*, enjoying your leisure time while using a sensible amount of sun protection, and hope the price we pay later isn't too high.**

Some would suggest that a little sun exposure is like a touch of pregnancy, but I must say, despite the raised brows of some of my dermatologic colleagues, that a fulfilled life must accept some compromise. And as protective skincare becomes both more user-friendly and more effective, it will be easier than ever before to enjoy yourself safely.

SimplyAgeless411: What are the most important ingredients that a sunscreen must have?

Dr. N.L.: Products designed to prevent sun damage abound, filling shelves of drug stores, cosmetics counters, boutiques, and spas. You need these, but there are so many to choose from. To help create some clarity, let me run through the types of ingredients that most of these products contain:

Emollients: These inactive, moisturizing ingredients constitute the majority of any given formula (other than water). They give the product its luxuriant feel, and they act to provide and retain moisture. As important as they are, they are overvalued and almost irrelevant toward effective protection from the sun.

Blocking agents: These are the agents that you really need the most. Their effectiveness in reducing sun damage is expressed as the SPF, or Sun Protection Factor. Although some products are available with SPF as high as 60, the FDA does not recommend any listing above 30. (The rationale is that there is no significant increase in protection above 30, and that the higher numbers might lull the user into a false sense of "sun invulnerability".)

Blocking agents are of two types: Reflective blocks such as *zinc* and *titanium oxides* offer the most effective protection against the entire UV spectrum, and are effective immediately upon applying. On the negative side, they tend to produce an undesirable whitish metallic sheen, varying in appearance from a slightly pale luster to full Kabuki. Current formulas are much improved.

Chemical blocks, such as *methoxicinnamate, oxybenzone*, etc. These are completely transparent, and may be as effective as the metallics. They do require about 30 minutes before they become effective, so they should be applied indoors before getting out into the sunshine. Some purists prefer not to have any chemical blocks on their skin, although these agents have not been shown to be harmful in any way. Many sun protection products today contain *both* types.

Anti-oxidants and nutritives: It's safe to assume that some harmful rays will penetrate even the most scrupulously-applied defenses, and so these ingredients help to replenish some of the depleted healing resources. These include retinols (Vitamin A derivatives), ascorbic acid (Vitamin C), and other compounds.

New DNA Based Technology on the Horizon

There are some exciting new concepts in sun protection based on DNA Technology. Sun-induced skin damage is commonly mediated by injury to the DNA of the skin cells. You may recall that DNA consists of two strands (of nucleotides), the *double helix*. Radiation from the sun causes the two strands to link together abnormally with bridges called *dimers*. If left unchecked, these *dimers* may cause the cell to either die early, which would produce premature aging of the skin, or worse, to become cancerous.

A revolutionary new drug currently in FDA trials is creating quite a buzz. **Dimercine** contains an enzyme that penetrates into the cell and cell nucleus, and cleaves the unhealthful *dimers* linking the two strands, which allows the *double helix* to return to its pre-injury state. In clinical trials this amazing drug has been shown to reduce the incidence of malignant and premalignant skin lesions by over 65%: *I'd call it a wonder drug for the young millennium*.

Enzymes similar to *Dimercine* are available in some over-the-counter products. One of them is derived from blue-green algae, and its activity is actually *turned on* by the sun...a beneficial dichotomy: the very sun that causes the DNA injury also activates the product that may heal it!

SimplyAgeless411: Wow...this is great information, Dr. Leaf, thank you. With these tips we will certainly have a better idea what ingredients to look for in our sunscreen and we will be watching for the new developments with Dimercine.

Top 4 Sunscreen Products

We spent the next few hours polling other top plastic surgeons in Beverly Hills for their feedback sun protection. We stopped in on Dr. Cynthia Boxrud's Santa Monica office for her advice. Elected by her peers into *America's Top Doctors, America's Top Ophthalmologists* and *America's Top Cosmetic Surgeons* from 2001 until present, Dr. Boxrud told us one of her favorite sunscreens (she actually carries this line in her office), is **La Roche**

Posay Anthelios 60 Ultra Light Sunscreen Fluid. It blocks both UVB and UVB rays and its texture is weightless.

Other top performing sunscreens include **Neutrogena Ultra Sheer Dry-Touch Sunblock SPF 45,** which contains a sweat-proof formula with Helioplex, an ingredient that helps to further protect skin from UVA rays. Dr. Boxrud recommends **Aveeno Positively Ageless SPF70** as a good for year-around coverage for the face and body. **SkinCeuticals Sheer Physical UV Defense SPF 50** is a groundbreaking first-to-market matte fluid with transparent finish. This paraben-free, all-physical filter sunscreen provides increased protection in an ultra-sheer texture for all skin types, even very sensitive. Sheer Physical UV Defense SPF 50 offers the photo protection of trusted broad-spectrum, physical filters, zinc oxide (Z-COTE®) and titanium dioxide, and is enhanced by artemia salina, a plankton extract, to increase the skin's defenses and resistance to UV and heat stress.

Sunscreens in Oral Supplements

Researchers from the American Academy of Dermatology have recently explored combining vitamins E and C as an oral supplement to provide sun protection. Multiple studies suggest that this combination therapy is beneficial for photo protection.

Cutting edge science is starting to understand more about the mechanisms of photo-aging, one of the most damaging causes of premature aging. And modern science is also starting to produce products that use the benefits inherent in these natural sunscreens. For example, a new Omega 3 supplement recently introduced to the market includes lycopene as an active ingredient, as well other ingredients that bolster your skin's natural resistance to sunburn. It can also help reverse the effects of photo-aging.

The Skin Diet: Nourishing Your Skin with Vitamins & Oils

Skin nutrition includes a diet low in saturated fat and rich in fruits and vegetables, which not only keeps you healthier on the inside, but also protects your skin from cancer. Healthy fats, such as omega-3 fatty acids, produce the skin's natural oil barrier, critical in keeping skin hydrated, plumper, and younger looking. Load up on foods high in omega-3s, vitamins and antioxidants, including:

- Selenium -- Brazil nuts, turkey, cod
- Vitamin B-2 -- Milk, enriched grain products, eggs
- Vitamin B-6 -- Chicken, fish, nuts
- Vitamin B-12 -- Clams, liver, trout, fortified cereals
- Vitamin C -- Citrus fruits, red peppers, broccoli
- Vitamin E -- Sunflower oil, whole grains, nuts

- Omega-3s -- Salmon, flaxseed, safflower oil, walnuts

Five Nutritional Supplements for the Skin

1. Vitamin B Complex - When it comes to skin, the single most important B vitamin is biotin, a nutrient that forms the basis of skin, nail, and hair cells. B vitamins give skin an almost instant healthy glow while hydrating cells and increasing overall tone. Niacin, a specific B vitamin, helps skin retain moisture, so vitamins containing this nutrient can help your complexion look plumper and younger in as little as six days. Niacin also has anti-inflammatory properties to soothe dry, irritated skin. In higher concentrations it can also work as a lightening agent to even out blotchy skin tone. In one study presented at a recent Annual Meeting of the American Academy of Dermatology, vitamin B was shown to dramatically improve how the skin ages.

2. Alpha Lipoic Acid - A powerful antioxidant, hundreds of times more potent than either vitamin C or E, Alpha-Lipoic acid may turn out to be a super-boost for aging skin. What makes it so special is its ability to penetrate both oil and water, affecting skin cells from both the inside and the outside of the body. Most other antioxidants can do one but not both. More specifically, Alpha-Lipoic acid neutralizes skin cell damage caused by free radicals, much like vitamins C and E do. In one study conducted at Yale

University and published in the *Archives of Gerontology and Geriatrics*, researchers found that Alpha-Lipoic Acid protected proteins against damage by free radicals. Studies also suggest that it helps other vitamins work more effectively to rebuild skin cells damaged by environmental assaults, such as smoke and pollution.

3. DMAE - DMAE is a powerful antioxidant with a strong appetite for free radicals. It works mostly by deactivating their power to harm skin cells. It also helps stabilize the membrane around the outside of each cell so that assaults from sun damage and cigarette smoke are reduced. DMAE not only gives you a more youthful appearance by improving elasticity and firmness, it also improves the contours of the face, and makes your mind sharper. It also helps prevent the formation of lipofucsin, the brown pigment that becomes the basis for age spots.

4. 7-Keto DHEA - DHEA is one of the most prevalent hormones in the human body. It promotes improved immune system function and anti-aging effects, as well as enhanced energy and weight control. 7 Keto DHEA offers these same benefits in a form that does not convert into testosterone or estrogen in the body, which standard DHEA can. A recent study shows that it can increase the thickness and softness of the skin as well as improve bone strength. DHEA is naturally produced by the adrenal glands and circulates in the blood stream, where it is converted into testosterone and estrogen as the body dictates. Your body's production of DHEA reaches its peak between the ages of 20 and 30, and then rapidly declines. By the age of 80, production of DHEA is only 5% of peak. 7-Keto DHEA, is entirely free of hormonal side effects. It also improves how wounds heal, decreases chances of getting cold, flu and allergies and can prevent pain in the joints and osteoarthritis. Something of a miracle supplement, it also lowers depression and provides a general mood enhancer to give you an overall feeling of well-being.

5. Green Tea Extract – This supplement gives you all the benefits of 10 cups of green tea without the caffeine or diuretic effects. Green Tea is a powerful and natural anti-oxidant and anti-inflammatory that has been used as medicine in China for more than 4,000 years. Researchers at The University of Purdue concluded that a compound in green tea inhibits the growth of cancer cells. Additionally, a May 29, 2009, Mayo Clinic press release confirms that a chemical in green tea (EGCG) had anti-carcinogenic functions. Research also indicates that drinking green tea improves skin tone and lowers total cholesterol levels, as well as improving the ratio of good (HDL) cholesterol to bad (LDL) cholesterol.

Believe it or not, there are many people who are unable to tolerate the diuretic effects of tea in any form, so the extract from green tea is a nice alternative as a supplement. Just two capsules contain all of the same benefits that you would get in drinking 10 cups of tea. Green Tea Extract is also a potent source of polyphenols and two antioxidant compounds that are 25 to 100 times more potent than that of vitamins A, C and E, which protects fragile DNA and cells from destructive free radicals. Antioxidants neutralize harmful oxygen-containing molecules in your body called free radicals and peroxides. Stress, exposure to toxins and even the digestion of certain foods creates free radicals.

Chapter Eight

The Role of High Tech Ingredients
Nanotechnology in Skincare

Antioxidants & Skincare - What are antioxidants?

It seems as if almost every skin-care product now has an added "antioxidant," and many men and women want to know if they really work, or if it's marketing hype. An antioxidant is any substance that slows or stops free-radical damage to cells. Free-radical damage to the cells occurs when natural light damages skin cells and extra electrons begin "floating around" looking for a home. When those extra electrons find a home (often in a cell), they usually damage those cells when latching on. This then triggers inflammation and cell injury. Anything that slows the injury process down is referred to as an "antioxidant."

Antioxidants in skin creams

Many vitamins, such as Vitamins A, C, and E have antioxidant properties. Coenzymes, such as alpha-lipoic acid and CoQ10, also contain antioxidants as do many plant-derived compounds. More and more creams and cosmetics feature these antioxidants and there is good evidence to suggest that some antioxidants, like vitamins C and E in serum form provide significant preventive and repairing effects for sun damage.

Nanotechnology in Skincare Products

Nanotechnology has been in the news a lot lately. What exactly is it and how can it benefit us? Nanotechnology uses microscopic materials (approximately one-billionth of a meter and only seen under a powerful microscope) to create everything from dental bonding agents, to cosmetics to medications. Research in the medical field has shown us that nanotechnology can help with the healing and repair of skin tissue. With cosmeceuticals, it is believed that the smaller particles are more readily absorbed into the skin and can repair damage easier and more efficiently. It is believed that as new products are developed nanotechnology may be also be used to prevent the graying of hair and might eventually combat hair loss.

Nanotechnology is taking skin care and cosmetics to another level. It not only improves how well products work, but makes it possible for other dynamic ingredients to be introduced into the making of health and beauty products that could not be before. It allows nanoparticles in products to go deeper below the skin's surface to produce better results. Sunscreens and some anti-aging products are at the forefront of those products in the market that are the result of nanotechnology. Some of the most recognized brands in the world are leading the nanotechnology movement in the beauty industry. L'Oreal uses the technology in the production of its best-selling Revitalift anti-wrinkle cream. According to L'Oreal, Revitalift's results are immediate because the product contains "nanosiomes of Pro-Retinol A". Estee Lauder also has a number of nanocosmetics on the over-the-counter market, as does Proctor & Gamble, Shiseido and Duprey Cosmetics.

Because of the relative newness of the technology, there is still some concern about their safety with long-term use. The Food and Drug Administration (US) and The Royal Society (UK) have called for continued testing and transparency in the research in the use of the technology in the manufacture of cosmetics. Some nanoparticles have received FDA approval, such as zinc oxide and titanium dioxide, which are often used in the manufacture of sunscreen products.

Exciting new developments are emerging in the world of nanotechnology which will result in significant improvement in the quality of life as we know it.

Humectants - Humectants are found in most moisturizing creams and direct moisture from the air into your skin. For this to occur the air's humidity must be at least 70 percent – humectants cannot draw moisture from the air into your skin if the air doesn't have enough moisture in it. They also help attract moisture from the dermis into the epidermis. Humectants are helpful for skin damaged by sun, particularly the thick, rough, scaly skin often found on the knees, feet and elbows. Examples of humectants include Hyaluronic acid, glycerin, butylene glycol, propylene glycerol, sorbitol, sodium PCA, urea, panthenol and lactic acid

Lipids - Essentially, lipids are fats that don't dissolve in water. There are many types of lipids that occur naturally in the human body. Skin lipids constitute 10 to 30 percent of the top layer (stratum corneum) and form the skin's barrier to prevent the infiltration of drugs, germs and chemicals into the skin. They also reduce the loss of water in the skin, protecting our bodies from dehydration. Many skin care companies incorporate lipids into their moisturizing and anti-wrinkle products. The most commonly used lipids in cosmetic formulations are ceramides and liposomes, which will be listed as part of the product's ingredients if you look closely.

Liposomes - These are microscopic spheres with an aqueous center surrounded by layers of lipids. They were originally developed for the purpose of delivering drugs, vaccines and other substances to the body. In cosmetic formulations they carry active ingredients to the deeper layers of the epidermis where they are absorbed in the places that are most needed to keep the skin hydrated for long periods of time.

Peptides - Peptides are chains of amino acids that work much like hyaluronic acid in aiding the "communication" between skin cells. Rather than delivering nutrients, however, peptides encourage your skin cells to produce more collagen and elastin – the compounds that keep your skin looking (and feeling) youthful. According to many dermatologists, some peptides are better than others. Pentapeptides, for example, stimulate hyaluronic acid, which we covered earlier as a powerful weapon in the war on aging skin. Cosmetic companies are using peptides in their products to diminish fine lines and wrinkles. Peptides stimulate skin regeneration, but must be used in a high concentration and not irritate the skin.

Serums – Serums are different than the other lotions and creams in the anti-aging regimen because, unlike other formulas, they are comprised of smaller molecules so that the main ingredients are delivered deeper into the skin to provide more immediate results. Some of the most powerful and commonly used ingredients in serums include vitamins, peptides, retinol, CoQ10, antioxidants, hyaluronic acid, peptides, growth factors and other anti-aging ingredients.

Serums work miracles on the skin but they should not be used alone. Most serums do not hydrate the skin, so a good moisturizer should always be used in tandem. The moisturizer leaves an invisible film on the skin that acts like a seal while the serum allows the key anti-aging ingredients to penetrate deeper. For the best and most effective results, apply your serum approximately 15 minutes prior to applying your moisturizer.

Alpha hydroxy acids – Exfolliants

Alpha Hydroxy Acids are a key ingredient to look for if you want to improve the texture of the skin instead of just temporarily affecting the way it looks. Instead of a product that sits on top of the skin, alpha hydroxy acids penetrate, removing dead skin cells, revealing a fresh, new layer of skin.. They not only prevent clogged pores, they enhance cell renewal through exfoliation. They hydrate, increase collagen, and improve the skin's texture, making it more radiant. There are a range of alpha hydroxy acids to choose from depending on your skin's sensitivity level.

They have been around for decades, and are widely used as a key ingredient in skin care products, and in facial peels. The concentration of the acid varies from products between 5 and 15 percent, but even low concentrations can yield substantial results. Some over-the-counter products have a hydroxy acid concentration of 12% that will exfoliate the skin while you sleep. The men and women we've talked to who use these products are happy with the results.

Higher concentrations of up to 70 percent acid are used by dermatologists and plastic surgeons to produce more dramatic results. At this level though, which can only be administered by a licensed practitioner, the skin will initially be very sensitive to sunlight and be irritated. Those with sensitive skin should *not* use these products. Don't use alpha hydroxy acids together with products containing retinol. If in doubt, always consult with a dermatologist. The most well known alpha hydroxy acids used in cosmetic formulations are: lactic acid, tartaric acid, glycolic acid, malic acid, citric acid.

Chapter Nine

Rejuvenate Your Image In Style!

Are you tired of people treating like you are old, tired and out-of-touch? Do you feel young, yet look way older? Are you upset with the way promotions go to "younger" employees who lack your years of experience? Do you yearn to be respected and treated with more deference? Is the image you see reflected back to you in the mirror someone you don't recognize anymore?

You have worked hard to be healthy and vibrant. You are exercising, eating right for your body, taking good supplements, and sleeping better. You are weight lifting, doing cardio and stretching. You have never felt better. Yet every time you look in the mirror you see the same "old" you. Guess what? So does everyone else.

Just as it is our responsibility to be proactive about our health, it is equally important for us to take responsibility about how we look. It is up to each person to be certain that the image they project speaks well about them and accurately portrays who they are. Image is communication. It's one of our most powerful forms of telling the world what we are all about. Give yourself an image assessment. Ask yourself if you are communicating accurately with your appearance. Do people get who you are in 30 seconds or less? If not, time to improve your image. It may prove to be your best investment after improving your health.

Rejuvenating your image is crucial for two main reasons:

1) When people look at you, they must "get" who you are quickly. If you look tired and out of touch, you will be treated as if you are.

2) When you look at yourself in the mirror, you must see the confirmation of the internal improvements you have made. In other words, your external image should reflect the physical and even the metaphysical changes taking place inside. If you are feeling younger, your image needs to reflect that.

As you force yourself to modernize your visual appearance, you will start to notice that you feel more energized. That is because you are now beginning to physically manifest "growing younger". You look in the mirror and finally can see your hard work paying off.

The results are visible, to you and to everyone else. For example: you just lost 30 pounds, have added muscle mass and are really shaping up. But you are still wearing the same baggy clothing as before. You look in the mirror and feel depressed. It doesn't look like you are improving. No one else is noticing either.

Now you go buy some new clothing that is well tailored to show off your newly improved physique or figure. Suddenly, you want to exercise more, eat better and keep improving, as you almost can't believe how much better you look. Compliments start pouring in and you bask in the praise of your efforts.

By now you may be thinking that this is pure vanity. Pure egotistical vanity! Why shouldn't everyone improve their health for the right reasons of longevity, wellness and independence? We say, "Let vanity lead you!" Why? Because if you really look in the mirror, you will see if your body is aging well, if you're healthy, and what shape you are in. That is, if you really look. Vanity can lead you to wellness and to a better appearance. There's nothing negative about wanting to look and feel your best!

Dark under eye circles may mean you have sluggish kidneys and/or liver, or extreme fatigue. Adult acne may mean a hormone imbalance or sluggish elimination. Creppy skin may mean not enough flaxseed, omega 3/6 oils, and/or lecithin. Flabby muscles may mean you need to do weight lifting and eat more protein. You get the point.

Vanity means you care about your appearance. You look in the mirror and see what needs improving. Your body talks to you, cries out for help, and you listen. Vanity can be a great thing.

Notice we didn't say ego? Having a big ego isn't the goal here. Having a healthy body, mind and image is.

Vanity can lead you to take better care of yourself and that includes how you dress and groom. This then can lead to compliments, lots of lovely heartfelt compliments. And that, my friends, will lead you to wanting to keep that great image going. Having exuberant energy, vitality and no real aches and pains will keep you wanting to take care of your health. What a wonderful thing to get better as you age instead of falling apart as most people in this country do.

What is a modern image and how do you get one? There are many books written about image and dress. You can go to an image consultant or hire a personal shopper. But for our intents and purposes, we want you to understand the key components of a modern image and what it may take to get you one.

When wanting to look younger, your number one goal must be to bring the "sparkle" back to your appearance by adding back the "definition" that has been lost with age. You can do that through your clothing and style choices, haircut and color, eyeglasses, and accessories. Skin tone and good teeth are definitely part of the equation too. Grey hair can look great if your entire image is modern, fresh and sophisticated.

After the age of 35, most people get into a fashion/style rut. They find an image that works for them and then put their attention on other pursuits such as their career and/or raising a family. Soon their modern image gets dowdy and out-of-style. When a person finally realizes they look dated, it can be frightening to "go modern."

Most people want to look modern, but not too young or foolish. The goal must be to look fresh, vital, and age-appropriately stylish. You don't want to look like your raided your teenager's closet! Also, please don't be afraid to "get your sexy back". Sexual magnetism is extremely important to your success in life. According to Napoleon Hill, famed author of bestseller *Think and Grow Rich*, almost all famous people in history had strong sexual magnetism.

How to Look Ten Years Younger in Ten Days!

We have developed our tips to look 10 years younger in 30 days into two groups. One is unisex advice that everyone can benefit from following. The other lists are gender specific and will be addressed as such.

Tips for Both Men and Women:

1. Exercise 3-5 days per week. Even brisk walking will add a glow to your complexion and make your energy come alive. Walking for 20-30 minutes in the sun will give your face a healthy glow that nothing else can give you. An hour a day is optimal.

2. Whiten your teeth. Laser whitening is the most effective and fastest way to brighten your smile. However, even at home "white strips" is better than nothing.

3. Improve your posture. Most people tend to slump over as they age. Just by consciously standing up straighter, you will look years younger. Walk with pride and look people in the eyes!

4. Put more energy and enthusiasm in your walk, your body language and your voice. Try to move and speak with vibrancy. Stop sounding old and tired. Walk on purpose with purpose!

5. Get a facial: at home or by a professional esthetician. The idea is to exfoliate the dead skin cells off of your face and allow fresh skin to show. Follow this by a good moisturizer. Simply exfoliating and hydrating will make your skin seem years fresher. Banish the blackheads and clogged pores.

6. Update your hairstyle. Every two years you must update your hairstyle, if not sooner. If your hairstyle has been the same for years, you are most likely aging your appearance.

7. Color your hair. Few people look great in silver/gray hair. If you don't, you can turn the clock back by darkening some of your hair or by completely coloring your gray. Always choose a color that makes your skin look healthy and is close to your natural color. Hold the hair color swatches up to your face and see what it does for your complexion.

8. Clean up your eyebrows! Men's eyebrows tend to get bushy and craggy. Women's usually get over-plucked or are unkempt. Either way, nicely groomed eyebrows will open up your eyelid area and make you look instantly more alive and alert.

9. Update your wardrobe by adding some trendier clothing. Get help if needed to create your style. Everyone looks better when they dress stylishly.

10. Shoes and handbags are a dead giveaway for an aging image. Opt for modern styles and avoid being overly conservative. The right shoes will take years off of your look.

11. Get new eyeglasses and sunglasses that are similar to your facial shape: oval with oval, square with square. Try to avoid "frameless" style frames. We need more

color on our faces as we age, not less. Colorless will probably make you look color-less too.

12. Don't wear "worn out" anything! That includes your leather goods! The last thing you want is to keep sending a tired worn message about yourself.

13. Think new, fresh, modern, and stylish and dress that way!

14. Wear colors that flatter your skin, hair and eyes. Find out if you have warm or cool coloring. If you have warm coloring and wear cool colors, your complexion will look muddy and you will appear tired and drained. Wearing the right colors will take years off of your appearance.

15. Have your clothing tailored. Don't assume it will fit you perfectly off the rack. Fine-tuning the fit of your clothing can really make you look like you're on your game. Here are some of the things to check:

    - A strong shoulder line: makes you look younger, taking away a "round shouldered" look

    - Sleeve length, pant length, and/or skirt length are crucial: Sleeves: about 1-2 inches below the wrist bone. Pants: need to have a full break if they are fuller legged. Little-to-no break if they are slim at the ankle, as they are worn shorter.

- Skirts and dresses can be any length that flatters your legs, but for day they look best skimming the knee, just above or below.
- The waistline of your jacket, pants and/or skirts and dresses must skim your waistline and flatter the abdominal area.

16. Hold everything you are thinking of buying up to your face and look into the mirror intently. You must notice how you look and feel. When you try clothing and/or accessories on, ask yourself:

- Do I look better? Healthier? Younger?
- Do I feel better? Happier? More confident?
- Do I look older or younger?
- Did my energy go up or down?

Tips for Women Only:

1. Get a properly fitting bra. The right bra will give you a youthful looking bust-line in your clothing, make your waistline appear smaller and help your clothing fit better.
2. Toss the "granny panties". Buy thongs or French cut bikini briefs and ban the back-of-a-barn panty line! Wear matching lingerie. You will feel more beautiful and sexy. That energy will make you glow more and boost your self-confidence and put a sparkle in your eyes.

3. Wear a beautiful perfume and body tightening lotion. Lotions that improve cellulite and have caffeine can really make a difference. This alone will make you feel more special and attractive in sleeveless clothing or naked.

4. Buy a pair of flattering heels. It will elevate you out of frumpy, dumpy mood fast! If you have to wear low-heeled shoes, make sure they are stylish and flatter the shape of your legs and ankles.

5. Pump up your eyelashes! Use eyelash-regrow products and eyelash thickeners. You can opt to get eyelash extensions or wear false eyelashes. Thick luscious lashes make every woman look younger and prettier.

6. For goodness sake, pump up the lips! Our lips shrink and shrivel with age. Buy a lip-plumping product to use before your put your lipstick on. If you can afford it, get your lips professionally enhanced.

7. Banish fat rolls, bulges and bra lines. You can do this by wearing fabrics that don't cling in the wrong places, smoothing slips and undergarments, and clothing that fits you properly.

8. Show off your best physical attributes in a classy way. Don't try to dress like a man, unless that is your gender (lifestyle) preference.

9. Make your hair look shinier, thicker and healthier. Get a hair-piece or hair extensions to have fuller hair fast. You can use hair regrowth products for thinning areas.

Tips for Men Only:

1. Groom, groom and groom more. Young men look super clean. Make your clothing, hair, and skin look as clean and fresh as possible.

2. Get a haircut every 2-3 weeks. Older men tend to wait way too long between haircuts. The newer looks need more upkeep, but it's worth it. Or shave your hair off if baldness is an issue. That can look great too.

3. Shave the back of your neck frequently. Young men don't have hairy necks. In fact, they don't have hairy anything! Shave, laser or groom your body hair too.

4. Consider using tinted moisturizer on your face for a sun-kissed healthy glow. This will make you look much more vibrant. Men look younger with a slight tan.

5. Dress to emphasize your shoulders and chest, not your belly. Select clothing styles that add width to your shoulder line and detract from your stomach, unless you have a six pack.

6. Wear a tank t-shirt under your other t-shirts or dress shirts to disguise "man boobs." New slimming t-shirts with lycra will give you a more sculpted look in your clothing. Then please, get to the gym!

7. Buy some silver jewelry: necklaces, bracelets and/or a great watch. Accessories can give your image an immediate update.

8. Upgrade your underwear. Toss the "white jockey shorts". Opt for boxer briefs or colored briefs.

9. Buy the right belt for your pants. Jeans need a heavier belt. Dress slacks don't.

Bonus Tips:

Put a "twinkle" in your eyes that says, "I am confident, I really like who I am, and I have a secret!! Nothing is more alluring. That's because when people feel like they look old and out of touch, they don't look people in the eyes as much. They stop walking into a room as if they are fully present. So own the room, have a commanding presence that matches your newly found confidence and image. If you don't have it yet, "fake it till you make it!"

Action Plan

for Skin Care

The basic skin care advice we suggest for men and women of all age groups is to: wear a high quality sunscreen with a minimum SPF of 30, eat a nutritionally balanced diet including lean hormone free proteins, dark green leafy vegetables, fruits and nuts, plenty of omega 3/6 oils, drink 10 to 12 glasses of water a day, exercise at least four times a week for one hour a day, get seven to eight hours of sleep per night, and take your vitamins/supplements.

Monitor your hormones and keep them balanced. Be certain your thyroid is healthy. Topically, apply a good quality moisturizer in the morning and at bedtime. Exfoliate gently two to three times a week. The three golden rules of skin care are: exfoliate, hydrate, and protect.

Here are some basic guidelines for each age group to go by:

In Your 20s: This is the time to arm yourself against the arrows that Mother Nature eventually slings your way. Research tells us that the aging process begins around 25 years old so this is the time to begin educating yourself about preventive skin care. Never go to bed with your makeup on and keep you body moisturized on the outside and hydrated on the inside. Invest in a good quality sunscreen, the best being ones that use zinc and titanium dioxide which are completely natural. Limit your alcohol and caffeine consumption. Don't smoke cigarettes or do drugs. Everything affects your skin, as it is your biggest organ.

Beautiful skin begins on the inside. Regular cardiovascular exercise, fresh air and good elimination (two to three bowel movements a day) will result in better skin and help keep acne breakouts to a minimum. Use a face wash that contains 2% salicylic acid to clear debris out of your pores. Choose a moisturizer that contains 10% glycolic acid; from a doctor's skin care line. Using a light nourishing serum before you moisturize will help your moisturizer last longer. Follow with a light eye cream that combats under eye circles and puffiness.

In Your 30s: This is the age when the face starts to actively age in ways that are both noticeable and frustrating. Action is key. In the mid to late 30s both men and women notice changes in the texture of their skin. The also begin to see enlarged pores. For women, these issues can be often be helped by supplementing their hormones with a touch of estrogen and progesterone. Both men and women should use high quality nutritional supplements to keep their skin young and complexions glowing.

This the right time to begin using more sophisticated skin care. Purchase products that have anti-oxidants, liposomes, and use nanotechnology: all with an emphasis on greater hydration. Cell turnover starts to slowdown. Therefore, more frequent exfoliation is highly beneficial. The Clarisonic cleansing system and/or exfoliant scrubs/pads or gloves helps to polish away dead skin cells. Minimal sun exposure coupled with continued use of sun blocks is ideal.

In Your 40s: Until age 40, your epidermis renews itself every 30 days. After 40, it takes about 45, 15 days longer. This slowdown in cell renewal results in a duller complexion and ultimately, fine lines. More aggressive exfoliation such as micro-dermabrasion and light chemical peels will be helpful in bringing back a more youthful glow. Start focusing on using more sophisticated skin care that incorporate lipids for hydration, medically driven serums that have vitamins C and E, retinoids (vitamin A), fruit acids, and peptides with nanotechnology. These ingredients will actually help to rejuvenate your skin with a noticeable difference.

Women should have their hormones tested for hormone imbalances, which can greatly affect the skin. Eating more essential fatty acids and healthy omega oils will also help. Focus on eating more regenerative foods than ever before, such as lots of raw fruits and vegetables. Aim for sufficient deep restful sleep, rest, and meditation, yoga, exercise and good nutrition to help your skin look its best. Keeping your weight constant within 5 pounds will help maintain the elasticity of your skin. A younger face is a fuller face. Having very low body fat, below 18 percent at this age will actually make your face look older and more tired. Estrogen enhances hyaluronic acid production, which plumps up the skin. It is also stored in fat; therefore severe dieters will look older, faster.

In Your 50s And Beyond: Vera Brown, renowned esthetician, is famous for saying that "By 30 you have the face you've earned and by 50 you have the face you deserve!" No amount of face creams or scrubs will make up for an angry mean spirited personality. Over 50, who you are will shine through in your face. Menopause can wreak havoc on our skin, making it dry up and sag. It is imperative to get your hormones balanced or you will most likely "age overnight". Facials, sophisticated skin care and laser treatments will all help, as will injectable fillers. However, topical solutions will never address the underlying cause of skin aging as will HRT.

If your thyroid levels are too low, your skin will become dry and flaky. Dry skin get more sensitive and can look red, rashy and leathery. Estrogen affects the collagen and elastin levels of the skin as well as hyaluronic acid production. Topically applied plant estrogens stop being effective and estrogen replacement therapy is the answer for most women after entering menopause and beyond to keep their skin plump and hydrated. Low testosterone levels causes thinning and sagging of the skin. Early hormone related bone loss also affects one's facial structure. Women who use estrogen and testosterone in conjunction with total bio-identical natural hormone replacement therapy maintain much softer, more youthful complexions. Balancing your entire hormonal symphony will be the best thing you can do for your face, health and well-being.

PART V

The New Age of Vitamins, Nutritional Supplements, Spices & Oils

The Ultimate Health & Anti-Aging Regimen

Chapter Ten

Nutritional Supplements For Your Daily Anti-Aging Regimen

Do the supplements you are taking really work? Could you be putting your life at risk? What is really in your supplement? Are you getting what you paid for? These are important questions to ask, but many people down their daily pill without really having all the facts.

One hundred and fifteen million Americans take one or more of the 75,000 dietary supplements currently on the market. Americans spent $25 billion dollars on supplements in 2009. None of those supplements are FDA approved, because the FDA doesn't require approval or testing on any supplements sold to the public. They only get involved if there are numerous reports filed from consumers about adverse reactions. The rest of the time we're on our own to figure out if what we're taking provides the benefits its claims to, or has any side affects.

There are a minimum of 50,000 adverse reactions reported every year, some dangerous and even life threatening. The FDA does require vitamin manufacturers to list all of the ingredients of the vitamins on the label; however, they do *not* require proof that the supplement is safe or beneficial. The burden of proof is on you, the consumer, to determine a supplement's effectiveness.

The right mix of vitamins and minerals are a crucial component for total body health. They become even more important as we move into our 30s, 40s 50s and beyond. With all the conflicting headlines about vitamins and supplements these days, and thousands of products on the market to choose from, deciding which supplements to take can be a mind-numbing experience. *Are drugstore vitamins and supplements good enough? Are the more expensive vitamins offered at doctor's offices "better" and worth the additional cost? Do I really need to take vitamins?*

If you are able to eat all of the servings of fruits and vegetables that your body needs at every meal, and if that food is farm fresh, organic, and pesticide free, then you most likely do not need to take vitamins. Even if you do eat everything your body needs to be healthy, the soil is this country is mostly depleted of minerals due to over farming. So the iron that you used to get by eating one bunch of spinach you now won't get by eating five bunches. The Second National Health and Nutrition Examination (NHANES II) reveals that most of us don't reach those recommended daily allowances on diet alone. A survey by the group indicates:

- 92 percent of Americans do not consume five servings of fruits and vegetables a day
- 40 percent of Americans do not consume daily fruit or fruit juice
- 50 percent of Americans do not consume daily garden vegetables
- 70 percent of Americans do not consume daily fruit or vegetables rich in vitamin C

Plans are currently underway for the FDA to impose increased regulations on the supplement industry. Until then, it's up to us to do our own research. We've done a lot of that homework for you. We conducted our own research using very specific criteria that wet thought would be the most pertinent and compelling to you: *purity, quality and efficacy.*

We found that many of the cheap vitamins found in supermarkets, drugstores and online are severely lacking in absorption properties and contain a vast amount of fillers, which leaves little of the actual nutrient in each tablet. Additionally, we have been told by both doctors and nurses that when performing surgeries and bedpan inspections they commonly see undigested vitamins and can even read the brand names on the vitamins after they have gone through the digestive tract. These worst offenders calling themselves supplements pass right through the body without ever providing any sort of benefits to it.

Potency is another problem, when you have pills that aren't monitored by any regulatory body. According to Tod Cooperman, MD, president of Consumer Labs.com, an independent company that provides lab testing to consumers, many products on the market today are inferior and weak.

"After testing over 2,000 popular vitamins and nutritional supplements we found that 1 out of 4 of those products does not meet quality standards," he says. "They have significantly less of the actual nutrients claimed on their label. Another problem is impurities. Herbs like green tea, for example, absorb lead and other heavy metals from the environment. Many of the herbs and minerals we tested contained dangerous amounts of lead".

One test you can do at home to see if your vitamins are absorbing properly in your body is to heat a small container of vinegar to 98 degrees Fahrenheit to mimic the environment of the human body. Drop your vitamin in the container and check back in about an hour to see if it has dissolved. If it hasn't dissolved in the container you can be sure that it will not dissolve in your body or provide any nutritional value. The only exceptions to this test are vitamins that are specifically coated in a "time released" formula, but we have been unable to find any such supplements on the market.

The most effective nutritional supplements on the market today will have one or all of the following certifications clearly stated on the packaging. If they don't -- do not buy them:

- **Third Party Testing** – States on the packaging that the product has been tested and is 100% guaranteed effective by a third party laboratory
- **United States Pharmacopeia (USP) Certified** - The USP provides assurance to the consumer, as well as those involved in manufacturing and processing, that the quality and purity of the raw materials used are of pharmaceutical grade quality. A USP certification stamp should be clearly visible on the packaging. See www.usp.org
- **NSF Certification** - a non-profit organization that certifies supplements' safety. See www.nsf.org

Third-party testing and above certifications are performed through extensive review and analysis by state-of-the-art laboratories and highly skilled chemists and microbiologists with the knowledge and expertise to evaluate the composition of dietary supplements. Evaluation criteria include but are not limited to the following:

- ***Verification of the quality and quantity*** of dietary ingredients declared on product label
- ***Levels of active components/nutrients*** — must be within a specified range
- ***Disintegration*** — determines how long a tablet or gel cap takes to dissolve
- ***Hardness*** — Makes for ease of swallowing
- ***Friability*** — No one likes to open their supplements to find broken bits and pieces.
- ***Absence of key microbial contaminants and toxins*** — these include unfriendly bacteria, yeast and molds
- ***Screening for heavy metals*** — tested for lead, mercury, and other potentially toxic heavy metals.
- ***Ensure the product does not contain undeclared ingredients*** or unacceptable levels of contaminants.
- ***Demonstrate compliance*** with currently recommended industry guidelines for dietary supplements.

All the above criteria — and more — must be met for supplements to be effective. The bottom line is, when vitamins and nutritional supplements undergo these rigorous third-party tests, you can be confident of their authenticity, potency, quality and purity.

Professional sports organizations including the National Football League and Major League Baseball urge players to take

only supplements reviewed by NSF at www.nsf.org or
www.informed-choice.org so they can be certain they are not
inadvertently taking a supplement that contain steroids or other
performance enhancing ingredients. There is an area on
www.nsf.org called *"certified for sport"* that indicates which
brands are acceptable for athletes to use. For the average
consumer who would like to have their supplements tested by an
independent lab, you can go to www.consumerlab.com . You can
send them your supplements to be tested for a very reasonable fee.

We researched the above organizations and consulted an
independent research firm's latest manual, *The NutriSearch
Comparative Guide to Nutritional Supplements,* to find out which
brands of vitamins that can be purchased without going through a
doctor ranked highest in quality and efficacy under the most
rigorous testing.

The top brands are:
- Life Extension Vitamins – www.LEF.org
- Vitamin Research Products – www.VRP.org
- USANA Health Sciences - www.USANA.com
- New Chapter Vitamins – www.NewChapter.com
- Source Naturals - www.SourceNaturals.com
- Neutraceutical Sciences Institute –
  www.Healthyandorganic.com

- Swanson Vitamins   www.SwansonVitamins.com

Next in line are also top brands receiving 4 stars:
- Country Life Vitamins – www.CountryLifeVitamins.com
- Enzymatic Therapy – www.EnzymaticTherapy.com
- Nutriex Sport - www.Nutriex.com
- Thorne Research – www.Thorne.com
- Vitamin Shoppe – www.VitaminShoppe.com
- Julian Whitaker, MD. – www.DrWhitaker.com
- Jarrow Formulas – www.Jarrow.com

The vitamin and nutritional supplement industry is a multi-billion dollar business. There are hundreds of different types of vitamins to address virtually every aspect of the human body. Do we really need all of these? If not, which ones are the most important?

We interviewed over a dozen anti-aging/integrative medical physicians and asked them which vitamins and supplements would they want with them if stranded on a desert island. These are their collective answers, along with a list of other important vitamins, minerals, nutritional supplements and even spices that may not be in the Top 10, but are valuable and should be considered as part of a daily supplement regimen.

Top Ten Supplements for Ages 35 & Up

1. Multi-Vitamin
2. CoQ10
3. Omega 3 Fish Oil
4. Vitamin D
5. Alpha Lipoic Acid
6. Selenium
7. Flaxseed Oil
8. Probiotics
9. Olive Oil
10. Vitamin C

. Top Five Supplements 35 years & Under

1. Multi-vitamin
2. Omega 3 Fish Oil
3. Probiotics
4. Vitamin D (if sun exposure is limited)
5. Vitamin C

Additional Supplements & Herbs & Nutritional Support:

- Omega 6 oils such as flaxseed oils are great for the skin at any age
- Drink green tea daily or use flavored green tea drops in water
- Milk Thistle (to cleanse their liver)

- Dandelion Root (supports the liver, provides calcium and potassium)
- Holy Basil (for young women with mild mood disorders) by New Chapter
- Maca for energy and enhanced libido (especially good for men)
- Multi-Greens by Young Living Oils (supplements vegetables)
- Zico or VitaCoco Coconut Water to replace potassium and rehydrate after workouts or sports
- Pomegranite juice, Acai berry, Noni berry or other anti-oxidant juices
- Energy Smoothie
- Almond, Soy or Rice Milk
- Super Foods (organic vegetables and fruits) by American Botanical Pharmacy
- Multi greens powder like Orac-Energy Greens by Paradise (which has fruit in it too)
- Protein powder: egg white powder or whey powder (Jay Robb's is great)
- Lecithin Powder
- Brewer's Yeast from Lewis Labs (loaded with amino acids and protein) great for vegans or vegetarians. Fabulous for building muscle mass and endurance.

Nutritional Supplements For A New Age

Alpha Lipoic Acid - A powerful antioxidant, more potent than either vitamin C or E. Alpha-Lipoic acid may turn out to be a super-boost for aging skin. What makes it so special is its ability to penetrate both oil and water, affecting skin cells from both the inside and the outside of the body. Most other antioxidants can do one but not both. More specifically Alpha-Lipoic acid helps neutralize skin cell damage caused by free radicals, much like vitamins C and E do. In one study conducted at Yale University and published in the *Archives of Gerontology and Geriatrics*, researchers found that Alpha-Lipoic Acid protected proteins against damage by free radicals. Studies also suggest that it helps other vitamins work more effectively to rebuild skin cells damaged by environmental assaults, such as smoke and pollution. Alpha Lipoic Acid inhibits the formation of age-related AGEs (advanced glycation end products), which can cause a number of conditions such as high blood pressure and age spots. Recommended dosage is 100 to 300 milligrams per day.

The B Vitamins

The B Vitamins are important coenzymes that actually facilitate the breakdown of carbohydrates into glucose, which gives us energy. They are essential for the breakdown of fats and proteins, which aids the normal functioning of the nervous system, enhances muscle tone in the stomach and intestinal tract, and is key for healthy skin, hair, and eyes. Since these vitamins affect so many crucial elements of your body, a supplement that provides all of them in a single daily source (such as a capsule or tablet) is highly recommended. B Vitamins are water soluble and need to be taken daily. The B vitamins are important for the proper formation of every cell in your body, particularly nerve cells. This is why it is so important for pregnant women to take supplements that contain the B vitamins, particularly folic acid, and why a deficiency of certain B vitamins manifests itself first as a depression or moodiness. Vitamin B1, or thiamine, helps the body turn carbohydrates into energy.

Several studies have shown that the majority of patients admitted to the hospital for depression have a deficiency in the B vitamins pyridoxine and cobalamin. Taking a multivitamin or a B-vitamin complex may help with depression. Taking extra pyridoxine and cobalamin not only helps depression, but also fights aging and helps boost your immune system. Folic acid also helps your lungs, skin, and protects your intestines against infection. Taking high doses of pyridoxine, cobalamin and folic acid will also protect you from heart disease. Do not take more than 2000 mg a day of pyridoxine, unless prescribed by a doctor. The B_{12} vitamin is of note because it is not available from plant products, making B_{12} deficiency a concern for vegans.

Foods such as nutritional yeast and brewer's yeast, molasses, marmite and vegemite are some of the world's richest known sources of vitamin B_{12}.

B Vitamins: B1, B2, B3, B5, B6, B7, B9 & B12

Vitamin B_1 (Thiamine): RDA is 10-100 mg. Daily requirements of Vitamin B1 increase with diets that are high in carbohydrates and sugars. Vitamin B1 is a water-soluble vitamin that is essential for the breakdown of carbohydrates into glucose. Thiamine is also important for the proper functioning of the nervous system, as it regulates mental function, nerve growth and can help with memory. Thiamine is found in whole-grains, red meat, pork, liver, fish, egg yolks, green leafy vegetables, legumes, sweet corn, peas, brown rice, oranges, berries, peanut butter, and yeast. Thiamin is absorbed through the intestines.

Vitamin B_2 (Riboflavin): RDA is 10-400 mg. Higher doses are shown to reduce migraine headaches. Vitamin B2 is a water-soluble vitamin that is important in the breakdown of carbohydrates, fats, and proteins. Riboflavin releases energy from foods, makes many of your body's hormones and aids in growth and development. It is also important for healthy skin and mucous membranes, the cornea of the eye and the nerves. Riboflavin is found in whole-grain products, milk, meat, beans, nuts, avocados, green leafy vegetables, eggs, cheese and peas.

Vitamin B$_3$ (Niacin or niacinamide, sometimes also known as vitamin PP): RDA is 50-100 mg. Vitamin B3/niacin increases energy levels and is essential in DNA Repair. It helps the body metabolize food and makes for healthy skin, nerves and gastrointestinal function. Niacin is used for more 50-body processes, including releasing energy from food, making hormones, removing toxins and helping to keep your cholesterol within the normal range. Niacin is found in protein-rich foods, the most common include diary products, meats, fish, brewer's yeast, milk, eggs, legumes, potatoes and peanuts. If too much niacin is consumed, itching, headaches, cramps, nausea and skin eruptions may occur, so follow the RDA.

Vitamin B$_5$ (Pantothenic acid): RDA 10-100 mg. Vitamin B5 releases energy from food. It works with other B vitamins to help break down proteins, fats, carbohydrates, lipids and some amino acids. It also speeds wound healing; high doses of pantothine can reduce cholesterol levels. It is also needed to make vitamin D and red blood cells. Pantothenic acid is produced by bacteria in the intestines. It is found in liver, fish, chicken, meats, legumes and whole-grains.

Vitamin B$_6$ (Pyridoxine, pyridoxil, or pyridoximine, or pyridoxine hydrochloride): RDA is 10-50 mg. Vitamin B6 can help prevent heart disease and combat depression. It is needed for neurotransmitters, such as serotonin and may relieve PMS. Vitamin B6 is essential to breakdown carbohydrates, proteins and fats. It is also used in the production of red blood cells. Pyridoxine can be found in many foods. Some of the foods that contain it are: liver, meat, brown rice, fish, chicken, butter, wheat germ, potatoes, peas, beans, avocados, whole grain cereals, and soybeans.

Vitamin B$_7$ (Biotin): RDA is 30-100 mcg. High dosages, combined with chromium, improve blood-sugar control. Biotin breaks down the proteins, carbohydrates and fats your body converts to energy. Foods that contain biotin are liver, salmon, clams, eggs, milk, peanut butter and bananas.

Vitamin B$_9$ (Folic Acid): RDA is 400-800 mcg. Folic acid is produced by bacteria in the stomach and intestines and is essential to the growth and division of cells. It prevents birth defects and heart disease and may help prevent colon cancer. It interacts with vitamin B12 for the synthesis of DNA and is also necessary for the breakdown of proteins and the formation of hemoglobin. It is found in many foods, including yeast, liver, green vegetables, avocados, beets, orange juice, beans, and whole grain cereals. Women who are pregnant have an increased need for folic acid.

Vitamin B$_{12}$ (various cobalamins; commonly cyanocobalamins in vitamin supplements): RDA is 20-1,000 mcg. B12 is stored in the liver and may improve memory and reverse an inability to concentrate, or "mental fogginess." Cobalamin breaks down the proteins, carbohydrates and fats you consume to give you energy. It makes the blood cells in our bodies and prevents heart disease and depression. Foods that contain Vitamin B12 are eggs, milk, yogurt, chicken, fish and meat.

Brewer's Yeast - Body builders have been using brewer's yeast for years because of its facility to build muscle. It packs a whopping 16 grams of protein in only two tablespoons and contains all of the essential amino acids, 14 minerals and 17 vitamins (including chromium) that control blood sugar. It is a one-celled fungus that grows on molasses or sugar beets and is loaded with minerals, amino acids, trace minerals, protein, selenium, potassium and many of the B complex vitamins. "It's this variety and abundance of nutrients that have made brewer's yeast such an enduring supplement," says Michael Janson, M.D., president of the American College for Advancement in Medicine, based in Laguna Hills, California.

Brewer's yeast is available in flake, powder or bud form for dietary uses and is most beneficial (and tastes better) when not heated. It is excellent on cold or hot cereals or blended into a smoothie. If you have yeast allergies or are prone to yeast infections you should avoid it. You should also steer clear if you are on the monoamine oxidase inhibitors (MAOIs,) or are teaking

Demerol. Ask your doctor if you take any medications before adding brewer's yeast to your diet.

Coenzyme Q10 - CoQ10 is needed to produce ATP, which is the primary fuel for cellular function. It is also a powerful antioxidant and protects the body from heart disease and various cancers, controls cardiovascular conditions such as angina, high blood pressure and congestive heart failure. CoQ10 levels can naturally increase through exercise, but a supplement form means more sustained energy. More commonly referred to as Q10. Medical studies show that those who regularly take Q10 can help ward off heart disease, Parkinson's disease, and even Huntington's disease. Additionally, Q10 provides anti-aging benefits since it also works to eliminate free radicals as a potent antioxidant. 200-400 mg. per day is recommended.

Vitamin C - Vitamin C must be consumed in food or supplements because it cannot be made by our bodies. It is a powerful antioxidant for the immune system, tissue growth and collagen formation. It reduces the adverse effects of oxidation and premature aging and keeps blood vessels and capillaries strong, skin and gums healthy. Recommended dosage: 1000-2000 mg per day.

Note** According to a top anti-aging physician we spoke to, to test the amount of vitamin C your body requires, increase your dosage 1,000 mg per day until you begin to notice loose stool. At that point decrease your dosage back to the amount taken prior to symptoms. This is a good barometer to tell how much vitamin C your body needs.

Calcium - We've all heard how calcium makes for strong bones. But a lack of this mineral means more than weak bones. Yet only 21 percent of us are getting the recommended amount of it according to federal government statistics. Organs need calcium to operate at their best. Because of its effect on the metabolism, it is necessary for healthy weight. When you're low on it, your body thinks it is starving and so it retains fat. Calcium also protects against colon cancer. The following are recommended dosages:

Ages 9 to 18: 1,300 mg a day
Ages 19 to 50: 1,000 mg a day
Ages 51 and Older: 1,200 mg a day

Do not take more than 2,500 mg a day because of the increased risk for kidney stones. If you have hyperparathyroidism or a history of kidney stones, talk to your doctor before taking calcium supplements.

Vitamin D - Vitamin D is actually a precursor hormone — the building block of a powerful steroid in your body called *calcitriol*. It's been known for many years that vitamin D is critical to the health of our bones and teeth, but deeper insight into Ds wider role in our health is quite new.

Vitamin D works in concert with other nutrients and hormones in your body to support healthy bone renewal — an ongoing process of mineralization and demineralization. Researchers are discovering that D also promotes normal cell growth and differentiation throughout the body, working as a key factor to maintain hormonal balance and a healthy immune system. Calcitriol becomes part of the physical composition of cells, assisting in the buildup and breakdown of healthy tissue — in other words, regulating the processes that keep you well.

The human body can't create vitamin D on its own. That's where the sun comes in. In theory, you can make an ample supply of vitamin D with as little as a couple of hours of sun a week. You can also ingest D through food, especially fatty fish like wild-harvested salmon. Since many people are unable to get enough sun exposure or follow a diet rich in vitamin D, supplementation is recommended by most physicians at 1,000 -2,000 I.U. per day.

DMAE – As discussed earlier in the book, DMAE is a powerful antioxidant with a strong appetite for free radicals. It works mostly by deactivating their power to harm skin cells. It also helps stabilize the membrane around the outside of each cell so that assaults from sun damage and cigarette smoke are reduced. A

DMAE supplement will give you a more youthful appearance, making the skin more elastic and firm, enhance the appearance of facial contours. It also helps prevent the form of lipofucsin, the pesky brown pigment this the basis of age spots. On the inside, you'll find you have a sharper memory and a heightened ability to problem solve.

Vitamin E – Vitamin E is a powerful antioxidant that neutralizes the free radicals that cause tissue and cellular damage, which can lead to cardiovascular disease and cancer. Vitamin E keeps the blood flowing and clotting as it should and helps wounds heal. Some studies have shown that it can decrease symptoms of premenstrual syndrome and certain breast diseases, including breast cancer. Vitamin E also may block the formation of nitrosamines, which are carcinogens formed in the stomach from nitrites consumed in the diet. One study shows that a liquid form of the vitamin also improves the clarity of the lens of the eye, which could reduce the chance of cataracts later on. 100 IU or more of Vitamin E a day should be an easy addition to your daily supplement intake. If you have a pre-existing heart disease, 800 to 1600 IU is recommended. Check with your doctor, though. Because E is fat-soluble, it is stored and so your body can "overdose," in which the vitamin becomes toxic.

Food Sources of Vitamin E
- Wheat germ

- Vegetable oil and margarine
- Avocado
- Whole grain products
- Egg yolk
- Nuts
- Liver
- Peanut butter

Some people prefer cold-water dispersible dry powder vitamin E supplements in the form of alpha tocopheryl succinate or acetate because the cold-water dispersible forms are efficiently absorbed even when taken on an empty stomach or with a low-fat meal. They are also twice as expensive as the oil-based Vitamin E. Note that the non-cold water dispersible (oil) forms of vitamin E may be poorly absorbed unless taken with several grams of fats or oils. Cold-water dispersible vitamin E, whether in a succinate or acetate form, always comes in a white dry powder, while noncold-water dispersible natural and synthetic acetate forms of vitamin E are always in thick brown oil.

Omega 3 Fish Oils - In addition to eating fish a few times each week, we should all be taking supplemental fish oil, which is a rich source of the omega-3 fatty acids (EPA) eicosapatentaenoic acid and (DHA) docosahexaenoic acid. EPA and DHA are precursors to chemicals in the body that help reduce inflammation. Omega-3's have been linked with prevention and treatment of a whole host of health problems, including: heart disease, stroke, high cholesterol, high blood pressure, diabetes, obesity, arthritis, osteoporosis, Schizophrenia, Alzheimer's, ADHD and skin disorders. Omega-3-rich fish oil supplements do double-duty in protecting the heart and blood vessels by bringing triglyceride levels down (the "bad" cholesterol) while at the same time increasing HDL (the "good' cholesterol).

Scientists have yet to work out many of the details about how omega-3s work their magic, but inflammation is one clue, at least for some conditions. Some studies have found lower blood levels of omega-3s in adults with Alzheimer's and kids with ADHD than in comparable groups without those problems. The United States does not yet have guidelines for DHA or EPA, and consensus among nutrition experts is elusive. But specialty groups, some governmental agencies and individual experts have started to take a stand on the daily amounts needed.

For healthy adults without major medical issues, the European Food Safety Agency recommends a daily dose of 250 milligrams of combined EPA and DHA, while the National Heart Foundation of Australia suggests 500 milligrams. A NATO workshop recommended 800 milligrams per day. EPA and DHA are often taken, and measured, together.

People with heart disease, according to the American Heart

Association, should get 1 gram of EPA and DHA a day. People with high triglycerides should take 2 to 4 grams under a doctor's supervision.

Pregnant and breast-feeding women should focus on DHA, aiming for at least 200 to 300 milligrams a day, according to several expert groups. "If they don't eat fish, women should take fish oil pills or supplements that have a 3-to-1 ratio of DHA to EPA," says nutritional scientist Bruce Holub of the University of Guelph in Ontario and executive director of the DHA/EPA Omega-3 Institute there. That's the same ratio found naturally in fish, he says, and getting too much EPA compared to DHA during pregnancy might diminish DHA's benefits. A 100-gram serving of salmon, for example, may contain 400 milligrams to more than a gram of DHA, and from less than 200 milligrams of EPA to more than 800 milligrams.

To be sure of what you're getting, especially if you're not a big fish eater, it might be easiest to go for fish oil pills, supplements or fortified foods. Supermarkets now carry eggs, yogurt, milk, juice, margarine, bread and other foods boosted with omega-3s.

With fish oil pills, look for varieties that are as concentrated as possible. Most are made from anchovies and other small fish that don't spend long in the ocean, but if you're worried about mercury or other contaminants, the Environmental Defense Fund offers a guide to brands online at www.EDF.org. Vegetarians can get the same benefits from algae-based supplements, which are also the kind that appear in some infant formulas.

For babies who aren't breast-feeding, doctors recommend formula fortified with DHA — as many studies show benefit and none show harm. Whatever your age or ethical beliefs, the bottom line is that you should get omega-3s however you can. This holds true for boys, girls, men and women.

Grape Seed Extract – Grape Seed Extract is a powerful free radical scavenger. It promotes healthy cell growth, reduces inflammation, increases blood vessel strength and elasticity and protects against heart disease, strokes and cancer. It removes "amyloid", a factor in Alzheimer's disease and age spots on the skin, it aids in collagen repair and reverses the appearance aging and helps protect liver and kidney cells. Grape Seed Extract is a more powerful antioxidant than vitamin E, vitamin C, or beta-carotene. Recent studies have shown this extract to be 20 times more effective than vitamin C and 50 times more effective than vitamin E at scavenging free radicals. Recommended dosage: 50-100 mg. per day

Green Tea Extract - No other food or drink has been reported to have as many health benefits as green tea. It's been used medicinally in in China for at least 4,000 years. In fact the ancient

Chinese proverb says, "better to be deprived of food for 3 days than tea for one".

Green Tea's contains a high amount of antioxidant compounds such as epigallocatechin gallate (EGCG) and catechins, which act as anti-inflammatories, support heart health, inhibit cell damage, protect against UV rays, can mimic insulin when the body needs it, builds bones and controls how and when the body produces heat. Green tea extracts have been shown to have more health benefits than an equal amount of black tea . Green tea extracts have more catechins than black tea, due mainly to its EGCG content, which has been shown to prevent LDL cholesterol oxidation and the lowering of LDL levels. This may help to explain the" Japanese Paradox" where the heart health of Japanese men is exceptionally high, even though approximately 75 percent of them are smokers.

If green tea doesn't agree with you because of its diuretic affects, a supplement of the extract is nice alternative without the caffeine or the increased need to run to the bathroom.

Glutathione – Glutathione is one of the body's main built-in antioxidants. The body makes it naturally from three amino acids: cysteine, glycine, and glutamic acid. Glutathione works in harmony with vitamin C and vitamin E to recycle these nutrients and helps with the removal of toxic metals, improves lung and liver function, boosts immunity and repairs tissues. It also has a direct correlation to how the body ages. Recommended dosages for healthy individuals over 50 is 100 mg per day and 200 mg per day for people over 70.

Krill Oil - is a higher grade of fish oil. It is a shrimp-like crustacean eaten by the blue whale in the oceans of Antarctica. For those concerned about the preservation of our environment, krill are one of the largest masses on the planet and are not in danger of extinction. Krill oil contains all of the same essential fatty acids of fish oil like DHA and EPA, but it also possesses powerful antioxidants called astaxanthin, along with vitamins A and E.

L-Carnitine – Carnitine is a naturally occurring molecule that transports fatty acids across the membranes of the mitochondria, the energy powerhouses of the cells, so they can be burned as fuel to generate ATP. It also benefits brain activity and mental function. L-Carnitine works synergistically with Alpha Lipic Acid to rejuvenate aging mitochondria. Recommended dosages range from 300 mg. per day to 1,000 mg. per day.

Lecithin - Lecithin is an emulsifier and has many medicinal purposes, primarily from phosphatidylcholine (PC), its the main ingredient. Once PC is ingested from lecithin-containing foods or supplements, it is broken down by the body into choline, which is vital for proper brain function. It is often used to improve memory for those who have brain function-related problems such as Alzheimer's, amnesia or dementia and has been shown to generate great alertness in elderly people. Studies have shown that people taking lecithin have significant improvement in memory test scores and fewer memory lapses than those who took the placebos.

Lecithin can also help your body in how it absorbs vitamins A, D and E, and you only need about 30 to 50 grams a day to get the full benefits. This amount can easily be found in egg yoke, wheat germ, soybeans, fish, legumes, peanuts, whole grains and yeast. Lecithin is also found in cabbage, cauliflower, chickpeas, green beans, lentils, corn, split peas, calves' liver, and brewer's yeast. Supplements are available in powder or granular form that can be added to food. It can also be taken in capsule form. It is recommended that the elderly take a 1,200 mg capsule before each meal to help digest fats easier. Both soy lecithin and egg lecithin products are available.

Not All Lecithins are Created Equal.

The potency and efficacy of lecithin is determined by its phosphatidyl content. A high quality product would have at least 97 percent phosphatides and be derived from non-genetically modified soybeans. Eating less animal fat also raises lecithin levels.

Fat Breakdown in Lecithin

By far, the most popular and established health benefit of lecithin is how it breaks down fat in the body. Though not considered an essential nutrient, it facilitates the quick and efficient utilization of fats in the body. Lecithin has also been discovered to help prevent gallstones and promote gallbladder health, and has also been used to boost physical performance in endurance sports. For decades now, it has been popular for treating patients with high cholesterol and has been said to prevent the build-up of fats and bad cholesterol in the walls of the heart, the arteries and the veins, promoting better cardiovascular health. For this same reason, lecithin can prevent cirrhosis in the liver by dispersing fat and breaking it down so it doesn't build up in the liver. This fat fighting characteristic makes it appealing for weight loss also.

"Lecithin has a versatile function in life," explains Dr. N.A. Ferri, MD. "It is an extremely important factor in the digestion and oxidation of fats, thus creating more muscle and glandular activity, resulting in greater body exertion and less fat accumulations. Lecithin is essential not only for tissue integrity of the nervous and glandular system in all living cells, but has been regarded as also the most effective generator and regenerator of great physical, mental and glandular activity. Shattered nerves, depleted brain power, waning activity of vital glands, find in lecithin, especially in the cellular structure of the nervous system and endocrine glands a source of dynamic energy."

Besides reducing the cholesterol level in the blood, there is mounting scientific evidence to suggest several other benefits from lecithin. It has been suggested that its intake in sufficient amounts can help rebuild those cells and organs that need it. Lecithin helps to maintain their health once they are repaired. It may mean that a deficiency of lecithin in the diet may be one of the causes of aging and that its use may be beneficial in retarding the aging process.

Thinking Younger

In his book *The Years Between 75 and 90*, Edward R. Hewith says that older adults can process foods much like younger adults if lecithin is part of their diet.

"With older people the fats remain high in the blood for from five to seven hours and in some cases as long as 20 hours, thus giving the fats more time to become located in the tissues," he says. "If lecithin is given to older people before a fatty meal, it has been found that the fats in the blood return to normal in a short time, in the same way they do in younger people."

Use in Cosmetics

Lecithin has cosmetic effects as well. It has been found to eliminate the yellow or yellow- brown plaques on the skin or around the eyes caused by fatty deposits. It keeps skin moist and can provide relief for feet that are dry and cracked. Lecithin was used in Germany 30 years ago as a restorative of sexual powers, for glandular exhaustion and nervous and mental disorders. Seminal fluid is rich in lecithin. Because of its loss from the body, men especially need to add a supplement. Its use is also considered valuable in minimizing pre-menstrual and menopausal tension. It is a natural tranquilizer, which is beneficial in nervous exhaustion and can help repair the adrenal glands.

Today's average diet however, does not provide enough lecithin to successfully protect or cells and allow lecithin to reap its benefits. As a result, lecithin supplementation is necessary for overall health and prevention of many conditions and diseases. Of its many benefits, lecithin has been proven to decrease cholesterol, promote cardiovascular health, restore damaged livers and improve the brain's memory function.

Lycopene - This natural red pigment is found in tomatoes and other red fruits, and is a powerful cancer fighter. New studies show that taking this supplement provides extra sun protection for the skin. Recommended dosage: 15 mg per day.

Magnesium - Magnesium builds proteins, releases energy stored in muscles and regulates body temperature. Researchers at MIT have also discovered it has properties to sustain strong memory well past middle age. Magnesium regulates the brain receptors important for learning and memory, and enhances the "plasticity" (ability to change) in the brain that keeps the neurons active and the synapses firing. Loss of plasticity is the root cause of the "forgetfulness" of older people. Magnesium can also increase the elasticity in the bones, and it partners with more than 300 enzymes in the body to give to better synthesize fat, protein and nucleic acids.

Adults should take 350 mg a day , easily found in dark green, leafy vegetables. But studies show that as many as half of all Americans don't get enough magnesium in their diets.

Melatonin - this is widely used now as a natural sleep aid, and for good reason. Melatonin is a hormone produced in the pineal gland found in the recesses of your brain, and it is crucial to getting deep, restorative sleep. Triggered by the daily cycle of sunlight and darkness, melatonin levels start to rise in the evening, crest around midnight and decrease toward morning so, ideally, you awaken refreshed. As with other hormones, melatonin production decreases as we get older. By the time you reach 60, melatonin levels are half what they were at 25, so it's no wonder more than half the U.S. population over 60 complains of sleep disorders.

A melatonin supplement can make a remarkable difference in your sleep, but it has also been proven to be a powerful antioxidant that may protect against certain cancers, particularly breast cancer. It also plays a key role in the overall aging process and may help retard brain aging.

When melatonin is used exclusively for its anti-aging properties, the suggested dosage is 0.1 to 0.5 milligrams under the tongue about a half-hour before going to bed at night. A study of patients over the age of 55 published in the *American Journal of Medicine in 2004* found that melatonin significantly improved quality of sleep. It has also been found to relieve symptoms of jet lag in people traveling across time zones. Taking 1 to 3 milligrams at bedtime on the first few nights at your destination can help reset your body's internal clock to the new location.

Multi-Vitamin - A Harvard study published last year in the *Journal of the American Medical Association* reviewed 30 years of supplement studies and concluded that when taken daily, multivitamins can help prevent heart disease, cancer, and osteoporosis. Experts agree that they are an effective and inexpensive way to stay well. To help you choose a high-quality vitamin that meets your needs, we gathered this advice from six supplement experts.

Demand 100 Percent of Vitamins - When you look at the "Supplement Facts" panel on the label, you should see at least 100 percent of the recommended daily allowance of some important vitamins, especially B6, B12, C, D, and E and folic acid.

Be Mindful of Minerals - While you should expect your multi to offer 100 percent or more of certain vitamins, this doesn't necessarily hold true for minerals. If you do see 100 percent of the daily value of most minerals on the label, you'll probably also see that you need to take several pills a day. That's because some minerals, like calcium and magnesium, are so bulky that manufacturers could never fit your entire daily dose in one pill.

Don't Overdo Vitamin A - Choose a supplement that contains no more than 5,000 IU of vitamin A.

Watch Out for Iron - If you're a man or a post-menopausal woman, take a multivitamin that's iron-free.

Seek Out Simplicity - Some supplement manufacturers include herbs like black cohosh or nonessential nutrients like para-aminobenzoic acid (PABA) in their multivitamins. You're better off choosing a supplement that doesn't include these extra ingredients.

Find the Small Print - Skip any multivitamin that doesn't have an expiration date or lot or batch number on the label. The expiration date matters because vitamins and minerals can degrade over time. Lot or batch numbers mean that the company tracks the supplements it makes and can recall one quickly if there is a problem with the product or its ingredients.

Read the Label - Important to search the label for a statement of what the multivitamin *doesn't* contain, like artificial colors, binders, corn, dairy, eggs, fillers, hydrogenated oils, preservatives, soy, sugar, or wheat. Allergies and sensitivities to these substances are common. If you have a sensitivity, these ingredients could cause inflammation in your digestive tract, possibly reducing the nutrients you absorb. If you're a vegetarian, look for a statement that the supplement is gelatin-free.

Get a Form that Suits You - Multivitamins come in several forms. The best for you depends on your needs. Tablets and capsules, the most common forms, are convenient to carry and take. Capsules tend to be smaller than tablets, so they're easier to swallow, but you may need to take several a day to get the same amount of nutrients found in one tablet. On the other hand, although tablets hold the most nutrients, they require binders to hold them together, so they may not break down as easily as capsules.

Liquids work too. People with poor digestion or those who can't swallow big pills may do better with liquid or powdered multivitamins (which you mix with water and drink). These don't require as much work from your body to digest.

The Following Is A Good Example of Essential Multi-Vitamin Ingredients

- Vitamin A (as Betacarotene, Natural Mixed Cartenoids, Palmitate) 5,000 IU
- Vitamin C (Ascorbic Acid, Ascorbate) 500 to 1,000 mg
- Vitamin D3 (Cholecalciferol) 500 to 1,000 IU
- Vitamin E (d-Alpha tocopherol succinate) 100 IU
- Vitamin K (as phytonadione) 50 mcg
- Thiamine (B1 from thiamine HCL) 25 mg
- Riboflavin (Vit B2) 25 mg
- Niacin (niacinamide) 25 mg
- Vitamin B6 (as pyridoxine HCL) 38 mg
- Folic Acid 400 mg

Resveratrol - the "red wine extract" is a powerful antioxidant produced naturally in plants in response to attacks by viruses or fungi. It is also found in small amounts in red wine. Resveratrol is one of a group of compounds that affect proteins in the body that help control aging. Studies at Harvard University show that resveratrol increased the lifespan of yeast, fruit flies and fish; a

2008 study showed it was able to counteract the harmful effects of a high-fat diet in mice. Experts consider it a fundamental supplement for any anti-aging regimen. 200-400 mg per day is recommended.

Selenium - Selenium is a trace mineral, found in the soil. It is essential to humans. Selenium is found in virtually every cell of the body, with its greatest concentrations in organs such as the kidneys and liver. One of its many roles is in metabolism. Selenium is vital for proper thyroid gland function and thyroid hormone metabolism. It helps cells convert thyroid hormones from their inactive form to an active form, which means it is very helpful in weight loss.

Selenium supplements come in organic and inorganic forms. Choose the organic supplement, as the inorganic contain sodium selenite and selenate that aren't easily absorbed by the body.

Selenium is also a powerful antioxidant that appears to regenerate vitamins E and C, and is often included in E and C supplements. When combined with vitamin E, selenium appears to have some anti-inflammatory benefits as well. It is also believed to prevent chromosome breakage, one cause of birth defects and cancer. It has also been used to fight viral infections and may even slow the progression of AIDS/HIV. Selenium also contributes to good health by promoting normal liver function.

A study of 1,000 men published in 2004 in the *Journal of the National Cancer Institute* of shows that those with higher blood levels of the mineral selenium had half the risk of developing advanced prostate cancer over a 13-year period. As a result, the National Cancer Institute has enrolled 35,000 men over age 55 to participate in the follow-up Selenium Cancer Prevention Trial, which is ongoing.

Other benefits of selenium include the protection against heart disease and mineral toxicity, as well as the neutralization of alcohol, smoke, and fats. It can help to increase male potency and it plays a part in the maintenance of hair, skin and eyes.

Additionally, selenium protects the heart, primarily by reducing the "stickiness" of the blood and decreasing the risk of clotting, which of course reduces the incidence of heart attack and stroke. Selenium increases the ratio of HDL ("good") cholesterol to LDL ("bad") cholesterol, which is critical for a healthy heart. Smokers, or those who've already had a heart attack or stroke may gain the greatest cardiovascular benefits from selenium supplements, though everyone can profit from taking selenium in a daily vitamin and mineral supplement.

Specific dietary sources of selenium include brewer's yeast, wheat germ, butter, garlic, onions, grains, sunflower seeds, Brazil nuts, walnuts, raisins, oats, brown rice, liver, kidney, shellfish (lobster, oyster, shrimp, scallops), fresh-water and salt-water fish (red snapper, salmon, swordfish, tuna, mackerel, halibut, flounder, herring, smelts). Selenium is also found in alfalfa, burdock root, catnip, fennel seed, ginseng, raspberry leaf, radish, horseradish, chives, fermented foods, sea vegetables, molasses, beer, eggs, kidney, medicinal mushrooms (reishi, shiitake), and yarrow. The RDA is 55 mcg for women and 70 mcg for men. However, for anti-aging purposes the recommended daily amount if 200 mcg to 400 mcg. A higher amount may be toxic.

Whey Protein Powder - The advantages of protein powder are endless. It is low in calories, so it boosts your protein intake without putting on weight. Drinking a protein shake after your workout builds muscle. Protein powders are made from a variety of ingredients available on the market but doctors will tell you that whey protein powder is "way" better. Use it in smoothies and shakes, sure, but it can also be added to sauces, hot cereals, yogurt. Several top trainers in Los Angeles have recommended Dymatize Elite Whey Protein Isolate as the highest ranking quality pure and natural protein powder available. It has 24 grams of protein and 2 grams of carbohydrates. We tried their gourmet vanilla flavor, and it is fantastic! This brand also carries the NSF GMP certification for maintaining the highest standards in dietary supplements.

The Spices of Life – Cinnamon & Turmeric

The 411 on cinnamon is in! Cinnamon is emerging as a true **Wonder Food** in terms of health protection. Who knew that it is also a natural appetite suppressant? Trust us, its bark is worth a bite. Here's the scoop...

Research has linked this yummy copper-colored stuff with lower blood sugar, cholesterol, and triglyceride levels, to name just a few. A recent study published in the *American Journal of Clinical Nutrition* found that adding a little more than a teaspoon a day helped tame blood sugar and curb the appetite. Cinnamon also contains polyphenols, antioxidants that create healthier arteries and reduce the risk of cardiovascular disease. The spice's delicious aroma has also been found to be energizing.

Cinnamon originated from tropical Asia, especially Sri Lanka and India, but as we know, it's grown in almost every region of the world. The spice, owing to its vast medicinal uses, had found a prominent position in traditional medicines, especially Ayurveda (the traditional Indian medicinal system). In some cultures, it has been used to treat diarrhea, arthritis, menstrual cramps, yeast infections, colds, flu, and digestive problems. Even in Western Medicine, it is now it is being used to treat obesity, respiratory problems, diabetes, skin infections, blood impurities, menstruation problems, heart disorders, etc. The most widely used part of cinnamon is its bark. Because cinnamon is nutrient dense, it is thermogenic, which means it naturally increases your metabolism. As your metabolism revs up you will burn more of the food you have already eaten as fuel, and store less as body fat. Cinnamon is rich in essential minerals such as manganese, iron and calcium. It is also rich in fiber. Plus it's delicious, how many medicines can you say that about?

More of the health benefits of cinnamon include the following:

- **Brain Tonic:** Cinnamon boosts the activity of the brain by removing nervous tension and memory loss. Research at the Wheeling Jesuit University in West Virginia proved the scent of cinnamon has the ability to boost brain activity. The team of researchers led by Dr. P. Zoladz found that people who were exposed to cinnamon were more alert, demonstrated better mental cognition and had more dexterous motor skills.
- **Blood Purification:** Cinnamon helps to remove blood impurities, and so has been an affective treatment for acne in some parts of the world.
- **Blood Circulation:** Cinnamon has a blood thinning compound that stimulates circulation, which can significantly reduce pain and send oxygen to the blood for increased metabolism.

- **Infections:** Because of its antifungal, antibacterial, antiviral and antiseptic properties, it fights external and internal infections and helps destroy germs in the gall bladder and bacteria in staph infections.

- **Healing:** Cinnamon can help stop bleeding and facilitates the healing process.

- **Pain:** Cinnamon is also an anti-inflammatory recommended for managing arthritis.

- **Diabetes:** Cinnamon has the ability to control blood sugar. Research has shown it is particularly helpful for patients suffering from Type 2 diabetes. Researchers at the USDA's Human Nutritional Research Center in Beltsville, Maryland, studied the effects of cinnamon on blood sugar. They found that a water-soluble polyphenol compound called MHCP, which is abundant in cinnamon, bonded with insulin to bolster its use in the body.

- **Best part:** Cinnamon is easy to add to the foods that you already eat and it makes everything taste better. Both ground and stick forms are equally healthy, but sticks have a longer shelf life (one year, compared with six months for ground). No need to grind your own: Pre-ground store-bought is as good as fresh ground and saves the hassle. Aim for 1/2 to 1 1/2 teaspoons (or one to two sticks) a day. So....spice it up! Try these tricks to get more of this nice spice.

Favorite 5 minute Low Fat Easy Healthy Cinnamon Recipes:

- Sprinkle 2 teaspoons of cinnamon and 2 packets of stevia or Truvia sweetener over a sliced apple. Microwave for 2 minutes until hot and crunchy. Top with high protein Greek yogurt from Trader Joe's. A yummy late afternoon treat!
- Add 1/2 to 1 1/2 teaspoons to **hot oatmeal** or **cold cereal**
- Mix 1/2 teaspoon into 2 tablespoons **peanut butter** and spread onto celery sticks.
- Stir 1/2 teaspoon into plain **yogurt**.
- Sprinkle 1/2 teaspoon over **sweet potatoes** or **carrots**.
- Toss 1/4 to 1/2 teaspoon of cinnamon over broiled **bananas**.
- Coat 2 cups of raw **nuts** with a mix of 1/4 cup honey and 1/2 teaspoon cinnamon and roast at 350F for 5-10 minutes.
- Shake three dashes into your favorite fruit **smoothie**.
- Sprinkle 1/2 teaspoon straight into your **coffee, latte,** or **cappuccino**.

Turmeric –Turmeric (*Curcuma longa*) is a culinary spice that spans cultures. It is a major ingredient in Indian curries, and makes American mustard yellow. But evidence is mounting that this brightly colored relative of ginger is a formidable disease fighter. One of the most comprehensive summaries of turmeric studies to date was published by ethnobotanist James A. Duke, Ph.d., in the

October, 2007 issue of *Alternative & Complementary Therapies.* Reviewing some 700 studies, Duke concluded that turmeric appears to outperform many pharmaceuticals in its effects against several chronic, debilitating diseases, and does so with virtually no adverse side effects. Here are some of the diseases that turmeric has been found to help prevent or alleviate:

- **Alzheimer's disease:** Duke found more than 50 studies on turmeric's effects in addressing Alzheimer's. The reports indicate that extracts of turmeric have natural agents that block the formation of beta-amyloid, the substance responsible for the plaques that slowly obstruct cerebral function in Alzheimer's disease.

- **Arthritis**: Turmeric contains more than two dozen anti-inflammatory compounds, including six different COX-2-inhibitors (the COX-2 enzyme promotes pain, swelling and inflammation; inhibitors selectively block that enzyme). By itself, Duke observed, curcumin, the component in turmeric most often cited for its healthful effects - is a multifaceted anti-inflammatory agent, and studies of the efficacy of curcumin have demonstrated positive changes in arthritis.

- **Cancer:** Duke found more than 200 citations for turmeric and cancer and more than 700 for curcumin and cancer. He noted that in the handbook *Phytochemicals: Mechanisms of Action*, curcumin and/or turmeric were effective in animal models in preventing and/or treating colon cancer, mammary cancer, prostate cancer, murine hepatocarcinogenesis (liver cancer in rats), esophageal cancer, and oral cancer. Duke said that the effectiveness of the herb against these cancers compared favorably with that reported for pharmaceuticals.

How can you get more turmeric into your diet? Add more of the spice to your favorite foods at home, drink turmeric tea or take extracts in tablet and capsule form. You can find them in health food stores. Look for supercritical extracts in dosages of 400 to 600 mg. The therapeutic dose is 2 grams of turmeric per day (1,000 mg 2 x's per day or 500 mg 4 x's per day) to achieve results as an anti-inflammatory. Higher doses are used for weight loss. Turmeric must be taken with food and may cause stomach sensitivity. Tolerance to higher doses can increase with time

Flaxseed Oil (Not just for beautiful skin!)

Flaxseed oil is considered to be one of the essential omega oils for optimal health. Most people know that it's important for raising "good cholesterol" levels, because of its high Omega 3 content. Flaxseed has been credited with everything from soothing bowel disorders, stabilizing blood sugar, lowering the risk of breast, prostate, and colon cancers, and reducing the inflammation of arthritis, as well as the inflammation that accompanies certain illnesses such as Parkinson's disease and asthma.

The big secret is that most people don't' realize how important flaxseed oil is for maintaining smooth beautiful skin. As we age, the cells of the skin tend to loose their moisture and get a creppy wrinkled appearance. It's as if we lose the "plumpness" in our skin. One day we look down at our forearms and thighs only to find our once youthful skin is now looking thin and aged. Flaxseed oil can help to reverse this "aged, dry, thin" appearance by actually plumping skin cells from the inside! No amount of moisturizer applied topically can do what taking the right amount of flaxseed oil can do. It will take about three weeks for your skin cells to "plump" up after taking a daily dose of flaxseed oil, so it's important not to miss a day. Most health care professionals prefer Barlean's Flaxseed Oil. Begin with two tablespoons per day for one month. After that, you lower the dose to only one tablespoon per day. It really helps if you exfoliate your skin in the shower daily, followed by moisturizing your entire body while it's still damp. Be diligent and you'll see a big difference!!

Take close-up photos of your forearms and thighs in bright lighting. After one month, take another photo in the same lighting. You will be shocked at the transformation and how much younger and smoother your skin became.

Olive Oil - is a natural oil that preserves the taste, aroma, vitamins and properties of the olive fruit. Olive oil is the only vegetable oil that can be consumed as it is - freshly pressed from the fruit. Olive oil is not only delicious, it is the highest source of monounsaturated fat (oleic acids) and polyphenols (an antioxidant). It is a prime component of the Mediterranean Diet. Studies have shown that olive oil offers protection against heart disease by controlling LDL ("bad") cholesterol levels while raising HDL (the "good" cholesterol) levels. Olive oil causes a reduction in the risk of coronary heart disease and also exerts anti-inflammatory, antithrombotic, antihypertensive as well as vasodilatory effects.

Olive oil is very well tolerated by the stomach and has a beneficial effect on ulcers and gastritis. Olive oil activates the secretion of bile and pancreatic hormones much more naturally than prescribed drugs. Consequently, it lowers the risk of gallstones. According to the FDA, consuming about two tablespoons (23 grams) of olive oil a day may reduce your risk of heart disease. You can get the most benefit by substituting olive oil for saturated fats rather than just adding more olive oil to your diet.

While all types of olive oil are sources of monounsaturated fat, Extra Virgin Olive Oil, from the first pressing of the olives, contains the highest levels of antioxidants, particularly vitamins A, D, K, E and phenols, because it is less processed. It has an antioxidant effect on the human body cells that stimulates bone growth, and calcium absorption. Most people do quite well with it since it does not upset the critical omega 6 to omega 3 ratio and most of the fatty acids in olive oil are actually an omega-9 oil that is monounsaturated.

When buying olive oil you will want to get a high quality Extra Virgin Olive Oil that comes form the first "pressing" of the olive and is extracted without using heat (a cold press) or chemicals. The less the olive oil is handled, the closer to its natural state, the better the oil.

There has been much fraud in the labeling of olive oil, which European nations tried to stop. We recommend you buy only *extra-virgin cold pressed olive oil.* It should be packaged in a dark green glass bottle to keep the light from oxidizing (spoiling) it. The best quality bottles will state the country of origin and the farm the olives were raised on, even the date the olives were pressed! The health benefits of olive oil last only one year from the date of pressing.

Unfortunately, few manufacturers put the pressing date on the bottle. Very high quality olive oil is expensive, but the health benefits are worth the cost. For maximum health benefits, use it cold on your foods and do not heat it or fry food in it as it destroys the enzymes and causes oxidation.'

Light and heat are the Number One enemies of oil. Keep olive oil in a cool, dark place, tightly sealed. Olive oil is like other oils and can easily go rancid when exposed to air, light or high temperatures. Do not keep more than two months after opening and store inside a dark cabinet.

Do *not* keep in the refrigerator. Although some people say olive oil can be kept for one year, about two months after opening, many of the nutrients weaken and start going rancid. So only buy what you think you will use quickly. After 12 months, many of the oil's prime healing substances will have vanished. All the vitamin E will be gone, as much as 30 percent of the chlorophyll, and 40 percent of the beta-carotene. Phenol levels had dropped dramatically, too.

Do not fall for the hype about canola oil being superior because of its high concentration of monounsaturated fatty acids. Olive oil is far superior and has been around for thousands of years. Canola oil is a relatively recent development and the original crops were unfit for human consumption because of the oil contained dangerous, fatty euric acid.

Coconut Oil - Coconut is highly nutritious and rich in fiber, vitamins, and minerals. It is classified as a "functional food" because it provides many health benefits beyond its nutritional content. Coconut oil is of special interest because it possesses healing properties far beyond that of any other dietary oil and is extensively used in traditional medicine among Asian and Pacific populations. Pacific Islanders consider coconut oil to be the cure for all illness. The coconut palm is so highly valued by them as both a source of food and medicine that it is called "The Tree of Life."

Coconut oil has been described as "the healthiest oil on earth." Coconut oil is a multi chain fatty acid. MCFA are very different from long chain fatty acids (LCFA). They do not have a negative effect on cholesterol and help to protect against heart disease. MCFA lowers the risk of both atherosclerosis and heart disease, primarily the result of the MCFA in coconut oil that makes it so special and so beneficial. Multi chain triglycerides, especially those in coconut oil, are not stored in the way that other saturated fats are. Rather, they are immediately metabolized by the liver and used as an instant and very noticeable source of energy. In fact, many physicians now recommend coconut oil to patients complaining of chronic fatigue.

Within the body, this ultra-beneficial MCT (medium chain tricglycerides) is converted into monolaurin - a chemical compound the body relies on to inactivate enveloped viruses. There are only a very few good dietary sources of MCFA. By far the best sources are from coconut and palm kernel oils. The saturated fatty acids in coconut oil are predominately medium-chain fatty acids. By way of comparison, both the saturated and unsaturated fat found in meat, milk, eggs, and plants (including most all vegetable oils) are composed of LCFA.

It is very healthy to cook with coconut oil, because it has mostly saturated fat, which means it is much less dangerous to heat. The high heats will not cause the oil to transition into dangerous trans fatty acids, as is the case with most vegetable oils.

There are a multitude of health benefits in coconut oil resulting from the presence of lauric acid, capric acid and caprylic acid, all of which have antimicrobial, antioxidant, antifungal, and antibacterial properties. Coconut oil has been extensively used in Ayurveda, the traditional Indian medicinal system for years.

Only recently has modern medical science unlocked the secrets to coconut's amazing healing powers. Published studies in medical journals show that coconut, in one form or another, contains myriad health benefits, including:

- A good source of "quick" energy.
- Boosts endurance for physical and athletic performance.
- Improves digestion and absorption of other nutrients including vitamins, minerals, and amino acids.
- Improves insulin secretion and utilization of blood glucose.
- Improves digestion and bowel function.
- Reduces inflammation.

- Supports tissue healing and repair.
- Supports and aids immune system function.
- Is heart healthy; improves cholesterol ratio reducing risk of heart disease.
- Protects arteries the atherosclerosis that lead to heart disease.
- Functions as a protective antioxidant.
- Protects the body from harmful free radicals that promote premature aging and degenerative disease.
- Does not deplete the body's antioxidant reserves like other oils do.
- Improves utilization of essential fatty acids and protects them from oxidation.
- Relieves symptoms associated with chronic fatigue syndrome.
- Is lower in calories than all other fats.
- Supports thyroid function.
- Promotes loss of excess weight by increasing metabolic rate.
- Reduces symptoms associated the psoriasis, eczema, and dermatitis.
- Supports the natural chemical balance of the skin.
- Softens skin and helps relieve dryness and flaking.
- Prevents wrinkles, sagging skin, and age spots.
- Promotes healthy looking hair and complexion.
- Helps control dandruff.

- Does not form harmful by-products when heated to normal cooking temperature like other vegetable oils do.
- Has no harmful or discomforting side effects.

The coconut itself is healthy, but it is the oil that is truly remarkable.

Coconut Water - is the clear liquid inside young coconuts (fruits of the coconut palm). With five essential electrolytes, more potassium than a banana, low acidity, and little sugar, it is an ideal health drink.

The "water" of tender young coconut technically is the liquid endosperm, rich in protein and nutrients, and considered essential to the human diet. Coconut water is one of the purest, most nutritious, and wholesome natural beverages found in nature. It is more nutritious than whole milk, and has less fat and no cholesterol.

It is a natural isotonic beverage that has the same levels as our blood (In fact, during the Pacific War of 1941-45, both sides in the conflict regularly used coconut water - siphoned directly from the nut - to give emergency plasma transfusions to wounded soldiers). It can keep the body cool and at proper temperature. It orally re-hydrates the body and is an all-natural beverage. It carries nutrients to the cells. It naturally replenishes the body's fluids after exercising. It raises the metabolism and promotes weight loss. Coconut water boosts the immune system and can help fight viruses, as does coconut oil (see our coconut oil benefits). It can also help to balance the body's ph levels and help combat fatigue. Coconut water contains more potassium (at about 294 mg) than most sports drinks (117 mg) and most energy drinks. Furthermore:

- Coconut water has less sodium (25mg), where sports drinks have around 41mg and energy drinks have about 200 mg.
- Coconut water has 5mg of natural sugars, where sports and energy drinks range from 10-25mg of altered sugars.
- Coconut water is very high in chloride at 118mg, compared to sports drinks at about 39mg. Our bodies need chloride to regulate metabolism and keep the acid-base balanced.
- According to the *Journal of Clinical Hypertension*, individuals with high blood pressure often suffer from low levels of potassium in their diet. Drinking coconut water regularly can significantly reduce your risk of hypertension.

People in tropical regions and countries have been enjoying this coconut water as an elixir for centuries. They have used the all-natural coconut water to refresh, refuel, re-hydrate, feed and maintain the proper nourishment and fluid levels in their bodies. Cultures throughout the world that use coconut in various forms have proven to have fewer diseases and ailments.

The benefits of coconut water are endless.

"Coconut water is the very stuff of nature, biologically pure, full of natural sugars, salts, and vitamins to ward off fatigue," says M. Satin, Chief of the United Nations' Food & Agriculture Organization. "It is the next wave of energy drinks, but *natural.*"

NutriGenomics: Made-to-Order Nutrition

Nutrigenomics recently entered the anti-aging medical landscape as a new nutritional paradigm that has scientists excited about its potential. Heralding a new era in nutrition, nutrigenomics is the science of using a genetic profile to develop a customized diet plan that will yield the most benefits for an individual, the idea being that not "one size fits all," not unlike getting your own hormones compounded bioidentically.

Nutrigenomics looks at the effect of nutrition on a molecular, genetic level. Eventually, you can eschew the Recommended Daily Allowance for diets made-to-order for your genetic make-up. Nutrition tailored both to your genetic make-up and occupation can also be envisioned. The diet for an athlete, for example, would take into account his or her genetic disposition to maximize its efficacy.

Nutrigenomics could also be used to boost health and longevity from an early age by testing the DNA of children and creating a lifelong plan for their sustained health and vitality. A single gene in some that predisposes them to heart disease, for example, could be identified nutrigenomically and a diet in folate-rich foods would be prescribed to fight the onset of such a malady later on down the road. Fascinating, huh? The advent of nutrigenomics and prescribed neutroceuticals can, and will, save lives.

What Are Nutraceuticals Anyway?

Nutraceuticals are the extracts of foods that have been proven to have medicinal powers on human health, particularly chronic diseases. Traditionally nutraceuticals were contained in capsule, table or powder forms in a prescribed dose. As their application has progressed in modern medicine, they can now be found in probiotic drinks and yogurt that are found in your local supermarkets alongside normally everyday versions of the product.

Resveratrol is one such example, probably the one most consumers are familiar with, as it has received a lot of good press in recent years for its anti-oxidants and anti-aging properties. Soluble dietary fiber products, such as psyllium seed husk for lowering cholesterol, soy, clover, and botanical herbs such as ginseng and garlic oil have been harnessed as nutraceuticals and appear in many products easily found on supermarket shelves today.

Nanoceuticals: The New Vitamin for the 21st Century

It's the latest coupling: vitamin supplements with nanotechnology. Manipulating molecules that are 1 billionth of a meter and integrating into traditional vitamin supplements sounds like an intriguing cosmetic cocktail, yes, but there can be too much of a good thing. Nanotechnology deals with matter that is smaller than 100 nano (from the Greek for "dwarf") meters, about 100,000th the size of one grain of sand. We're talking more than microscopic here.

The marriage of nutritional supplements and nanotechnology has produced what are known as nanoceuticals, which proponents claims endow standard nutritional products with a sort of superpower that makes them more active and beneficial by allowing the tiny particles to reach more areas within the body and infuse them on a cellular level. Some of the benefits of nanoceuticals reported by supplement makers include:

- More rapid absorption in the body
- Better metabolization
- Balance body's pH levels

- Increased energy

As an oxidant, a seek-and-destroy facility against free radicals. The elephant in the room here is the safety of such products, which is still unproven. Since the Food and Drug Administration (FDA) does not have the authority to regulate dietary supplements, the onus and social responsibility is on the supplement manufacturers to make sure their products are safe. Since nanoceuticals are such a new phenomenon, they have no proven track record yet. Their safety and efficacy as a supplement still remains unanswered.

Getting more of a nutrient may sound like a good idea, but many doctors advise to proceed with caution. Many nutrients taken in high doses that are above and beyond what is recommended can become toxic, so beware. The Project on Emerging Nanotechnologies has issued a report on their website, www.nanotechproject.org, which chronicles the FDAs inability to regulate supplements containing nanoceuticals. It is clearly be the subject of much debate, especially as the number of nanoceuticals grows and the technology advances.

A small but growing number of supplement makers have embraced nanotechnology. Their products can be found online. It's important, even critical, to review any available information on nanoceuticals and confer with a professional before starting any supplement program.

Action Plan

for Vitamins, Nutritional Supplements, Oils & Spices

In Your 20s – Men and women in their 20s should be taking a multi-vitamin to supplement their diet, along with omega 3 fish oils, probiotics, vitamin D (if sun exposure is limited) extra vitamin C and green tea. Spices & Oils: Cinnamon & Tumeric, Extra Virgin Olive Oil & Coconut Water.

In Your 30s – Men and women should be taking their multi-vitamin, along with CoQ10, omega 3 fish oils, B vitamins, vitamin D, Green Tea , Rhodiola (for extra energy), selenium, and maca (for men).   In both men and women, because of the stress of careers and children, the adrenal glands become taxed at this age and need increases vitamin B and C supplementation. Spices: Cinnamon & Tumeric Oils: Begin taking flaxseed supplements and a teaspoon of Extra Virgin Olive Oil every day.   Also add Coconut Water.

In Your 40s – Both men and women should be taking a multi-vitamin, alpha lipoic acid, extra B and C vitamins, calcium and magnesium, CoenzymeQ10, Vitamin D, Green Tea Extract, Rhodiola (for energy), Vitamin E, Omega 3 fish oils, probiotics (for digestion), grape seed extract and selenium. At this point both men and women should also consider herbs such as saw palmetto for prostate health (in men) and thick shiny healthy hair (in women). Spices: Cinnamon & Tumeric Oils: Take flaxseed supplements and 2-3 teaspoons of Extra Virgin Olive Oil each day.

In Your 50s & Beyond - Both men and women should be taking a multi-vitamin, alpha lipoic acid, extra B and C vitamins, calcium and magnesium, CoenzymeQ10, Vitamin D, green tea extract, Rhodiola (for energy), maca (for men), Vitamin E, Omega 3 fish oils, Grape Seed Extract, glutathione (for the immune system), glucosamine (for joints & cartlilage) and selenium. At this point both men and women should also consider herbs such as saw palmetto for prostate health (in men) and thick shiny healthy hair (in women). Spices: Cinnamon & Tumeric.
Oils: Take flaxseed supplements and 2-3 teaspoons of Extra Virgin Olive Oil each day.

PART VI

Diet, Exercise & Nutrigenomics
A New Beginning

Chapter Eleven

Your Health is a Choice, Not Your Fate... *so Get in the Game!*

We have the capability, through our own actions and decisions every day, to alter our muscle mass, strengthen our cardiovascular systems, improve the functionality of our cellular infrastructure and brain cells, increase and improve bone density and skeletal structure, improve the texture of our skin, increase our energy and dramatically suspend the overall aging process of our bodies, indefinitely.

We can shape our physical destiny every single day of our lives. Considering how few things in life are within our control, it's amazing this fact isn't more appreciated. The bottom line is that, for the most part, being healthy is a choice, not a destiny predetermined at birth. You are in control of your fitness fate, not at the mercy of Mother Nature. So get in the game and do your best to win it.

There is simply no better way to achieve optimal physical and mental health and improve your longevity than with consistent exercise and a well balanced nutritional plan. We all know this, it's tried-and-true, the fundamentals of a flourishing lifestyle. Exhibit A: A Japanese study at the *University of Tsukuba Institute of Clinical Medicine* surveyed 33 different aerobic fitness protocols covering nearly 190,000 people to determine their effects on mortality. Those with a low fitness level had a 70 percent higher risk of death from any cause compared with those who followed a more robust fitness regimen. This shouldn't be surprising. There is overwhelming, empirical evidence to support that a sound life program of ongoing fitness and balanced nutritional plan can sustain life and ward off debilitating disease. Not participating in your own health leaves you at the mercy of chance.

A new age is here in the world of nutrition. Scientists, physicians and researchers have discovered that by understanding more about how each person's metabolism works through blood typing and/or DNA testing, for example, the better they can help us lose weight and keep it off.

It's a common observation in Los Angeles that the gym is "church" to many people, and they go to worship several days a week. We popped in on two of the city's top personal trainers to talk fitness religion and find out what they recommend to their clients to get fit and stay fit.

Matteo Vettorazzo, is a world class athlete who has won the title of Mr. Italy twice in recent years, (see photos at www. http://web.mac.com/mat71). He trains athletes for competitions, helps brides shape up for their Big Day, and the average run-of-the mill every day people who want to tone up and trim down. We sat down with Matteo at *The Meridian Health Club* in Century City, California, to learn about the new world of Nutrigenomics.

SimplyAgeless411: Thank you for sharing your time and expertise with us today, Matteo. After spending a lifetime in the health and fitness industry and becoming a world class athlete and trainer, we are guessing that you have seen just about everything and have a good sense of what works and what doesn't when it comes to diet and exercise. Why do you think some people find it hard to lose weight and keep it off? It seems like thin people stay thin and heavier people stay heavy…what is happening here? What would you say is the Number One mistake people are making?

Matteo: That's easy: The Number One mistake people make when trying to lose weight is to cut calories as their long term strategy. They have been conditioned to believe that the gateway to their ideal weight is a simple math equation…calorie intake vs. calories burned, so they begin slashing their calories from the average 1,800 per day down to 1,200 or 1,300 a day.

When you reduce the amount of food you eat your body goes into "starvation mode" and burns only what it needs to survive. Your metabolism slows down and your body begins stealing muscle tissue to maintain itself in what it perceives as a crisis. These people soon find themselves exhausted, drained, and discouraged. They hit the wall and give up after three or four days because they run out of steam. I've seen it hundreds of times.

While reducing caloric intake is part of a good strategy, there is much more to consider. First of all, I never ask people to begin their fitness program by reducing their calories. I start by visually evaluating their body type. Then, I take it a step further by asking them their blood type, which gives me a solid base to understand what foods their body responds to.

The next step is to identify what their body in its current state needs to function. I then speed up their body metabolism with what I call a "zig-zag" method. The zig-zag method is when I have them alternate days where they increase carbohydrates so that their bodies won't become complacent with one diet plan. This keeps a healthy metabolism and prevents them from hitting that dreaded plateau and losing momentum.

SimplyAgeless411: Can you elaborate a bit more about blood type and weightloss?

Matteo: Interestingly enough, 99 percent of the time I can spend five minutes with someone and tell you their blood type based on their body type and behavior.   There is actually a website called www.4YourType.com where you can order a home blood typing kit to find out what your blood type is. Knowing your blood type is not only important in identifying which diet a person will have the most success with, but it also provides insights into their personality and behavior.

For instance, in Asia, a person's blood type is commonly listed on their resumes because employers have found this information valuable when hiring for specific job functions. A person's blood type is also important when choosing a spouse. When you are dating in Asia, a potential candidate will ask your blood type as quickly as they will ask your age, your hobbies or your zodiac sign to determine if you might be a good match.

SimplyAgeless411: This is fascinating! Do the blood type markers "positive or negative" have any significance is this area?

Matteo: There are four basic blood types…O, A, B and AB. Os are the oldest blood type on the planet. They (both men and women) are "hunters." They are naturally strong with a lot of muscle mass. They have very efficient digestive systems…they can eat just about anything without ever getting sick, and yet, they are quite sensitive to carbohydrates.

Type Os enjoy and respond very quickly to a workout regimen consisting of intensity-heavy resistance training along with high impact aerobics and running. They respond well to diets like *The South Beach Diet* because it is based around a high protein and low carb nutritional plan. Their nutritional plans work best with a 40 percent protein, 40 percent carbs and a 20 percent fat ratio.

Type As, on the other hand, are at the opposite end of the spectrum. Their digestive systems are the most sensitive. They will have the most success with vegetarian diets. They usually feel best on a diet of soy proteins, grains, and organic vegetables. They also prefer more low-key forms of exercise such as yoga, Pilates, walking and resistance training using lighter weights with more repetitions. Type As like spinning classes and low-impact aerobic classes as well.

Blood type Bs are all about balance. Unlike Os and As, they are a balance between the two types. Like Type Os, they have a very efficient digestive system and can eat a wide variety of foods in moderation, but they seem to be sensitive to wheat, corn, and lentils.

Additionally, Bs seem to prefer a more moderate exercise plan such as resistance training with light weights, yoga, biking and walking. Type Bs typically do well on *The Zone Diet* because it is pretty balanced. It has a ratio of 40 percent protein, 40 percent carbs and 30 percent fat. Type A's perform well with a composition of 20 percent protein, 60 percent carbohydrates and 20 percent fat.

Blood type AB is the newest of all of the blood types. It is even nicknamed "The Enigma" because there is not that much solid research on it yet. Their nutritional composition is a combination of the A and B blood types. Many ABs have a sensitive digestive tract and they do best when avoiding specific proteins such as chicken, beef, and pork. Seafood, tofu, dairy, and most produce work well in their nutritional plan. Their fitness regimen should be balanced and they thrive on moderation. They can go heavy or light with resistance training and they can do high impact aerobics or light yoga.

All of these diets such as *The South Beach Diet* and *The Zone Diet* are great starting points for people who are looking for a healthy nutritional plan. However, if you take it one step further and understand more about your blood type and body type you can zero in on which diet might be more suited to your body type and blood type.

The blood type definers "negative and positive" have no relevance in the nutritional plan. There's a book that you can buy that tells you all about it called *"Eat Right For Your Blood Type"*.

It recommends nutritional plans specifically for each blood type and lists which foods are the best and which foods to avoid.

SimplyAgeless411: Yes, that book came out a few years ago. There seemed to be a bit of controversy in the medical community about the fact that there was not enough data to support the eating-for-your-bloodtype theory. However, many people we have spoken to swear by this way of eating and have reported incredible results that last and feel great while getting fit.

Matteo: The science of Nutrigenomics is emerging with new technology around eating according to your genetic code. More commonly referred to as "The DNA Diet", people are on a nutritional plan that is in harmony with their DNA. Your genes play a major role in how your body digests and metabolizes food. Some people have genes that cause them to absorb more fat than other people. Some people have genes that cause them to store carbohydrates as fat instead of burning them as energy and some people have a combination of both.

For $149 you can swab your cheek and send a sample of your DNA to a company called Interleukin Genetics, http://www.ilgenetics.com. They will run a profile on your DNA and send you the results in the mail. The profile will not only define your DNA but it will includes recommendations on a diet projected to work best for you – low fat, low carb, or something in between.

These findings are just beginning to be embraced by our society and could revolutionize the way we eat. Understanding how your body digests and metabolizes food will tell you what you should eat to lose weight and stay trim. The DNA Diet is very similar to the program based on blood type. By having your DNA tested or your blood test taken, you can drill down to understand more about how your particular body type reacts to food and gauge which nutritional plans you will have the most success with.

Eating for your specific DNA or blood type will increase your chances of reaching your body's maximum potential. We are just beginning to get smarter about the world of nutrigenomics and understanding how our bodies work.

SimplyAgeless411: Can you tell us how to calculate the composition of our daily food intake? For instance, if our nutritional plan tells us to use the 40/40/20 split, what is the easiest way to measure and monitor that?

Matteo: To calculate the composition of your daily food intake you can purchase a device called "The Fitbit" (www.fitbit.com). It is new wi-fi technology that you wear all day and then plug into your computer to download the information. The product comes with software that allows you enter in your favorite foods and then provides you with the nutritional breakdown of calories, carbs, fats, proteins, sodium, potassium and much more. You wear the chip around all day and it will tell you how many steps you've taken and how many calories you've burned. It's only $99.

SimplyAgeless411: Eating healthy fats plays an important role in health and longevity. Can you tell us the importance of fat in our daily diet?

Matteo: Fat is the most vital macronutrient needed to sustain life, no human being can live without it. It's an evolutionary thing from back in the caveman days. Evolution taught us how to use fat, so there is no reason to switch to a "fat free" diet. Our brains are made up of a high percentage of fat—fats are vital for a healthy brain…healthy fat for a healthy brain. Fat is also the number one cravings controller. Interestingly enough, fat is the best way to keep your cravings at bay. If you don't eat enough fat you will be preoccupied with thoughts about food.

Sources of good fat include avocados, walnuts, almonds, pistachios and olive oil. Eating fat in combination with other foods (especially carbohydrates) slows digestion and signals the brain that you're full — so you will stop wanting more. Fat substitutes – what I call "fake fat" - trigger the promise of fat through enzymes in the mouth but never deliver. They don't break down the same way in the GI tract as real fat does. Waiting for the real deal, the brain continues to transmit a "still hungry — eat more" message to your stomach. The bottom line is to identify how much fat your body type needs based on your blood type or DNA test and stay within that percentage with good fats.

SimplyAgeless411:   Portion size is another key issue. Can you talk a little bit about this?   . How important is portion size even when eating good proteins…does it convert to fat even if we eat too much of the foods that are good for us?

Matteo: It's important for people to understand that what your body doesn't burn off, it stores. For instance, if your body only needs six ounces of fish and you eat ten ounces, your body will convert the remainder to fat. Even though it is a good protein, if it's more than the body can metabolize, what's left will become fat. The best advice is to keep your portions to the size of your palm, which is approximately six to eight ounces.

SimplyAgeless411: Thank you so much for your time today, Matteo, your insight into these new nutritional plans designed around our own DNA, blood and body types are truly revolutionary. We really appreciate your insight!

The Dynamic Duo of Exercise & Physiology

After our fascinating talk with Matteo we headed over to The Beverly Hills Sports Club to speak with Gerard Karsenty, a fitness guru to many top celebrities who has been training clients on both coasts for 15 years. He specializes in body composition, change and weight management.

SimplyAgeless411: Gerard, thank you so much for meeting with us today. What would you say is your basic philosophy about fitness and the role of weight training?

GK: Fitness and health are one and the same to me in life: they are inseparable. Fitness needs to be applicable to everyday life. The newer goal is to train the body from the inside out, not outside in. Movements need to be fully integrated from head to toe. Health is defined as the general condition of the body in reference to soundness and vigor. I believe that the greater your health and fitness, the greater your ability to live it well, pain free and with great vitality and longevity.

Weight training for decades has put too much emphasis on aesthetics, which has led most people to equate a nice-looking body with good general health. Nothing could be further from the truth. Weight training should be used as part of a *total* fitness routine, not the whole of it to look a specific way, merely to "be buff." I like to train people with the concept of working them out from the "feet up". The feet take the brunt of our movements. Then I address body alignment, core, posture, muscle strength, flexibility, mobility and neuromuscular strength and connectivity.

__SimplyAgeless411:__ In your opinion, what is the newer, more effective way to work out?

__GK__: I believe in "integrative exercise". Integrative exercise is working the body out in a multi-planar, proprioceptively enriched environment. In layman's terms, this basically means doing full-body exercises, from head to toe, as much as possible since that's basically how we use our bodies day to day. For example, instead of doing a leg extension that puts emphasis mostly on the quadriceps in knee extension, do squats instead. This exercise still puts emphasis on the quads, but it also allows for a more natural movement pattern involving most muscles of the body including the hamstrings, gluteal, adductor and abductor muscles. Core strength is needed and used and the entire body is working as a functional unit. And what do squats look like? Getting in out and out of chairs, something we do all the time!

__SimplyAgeless411:__ I have heard you refer to Absolute Strength vs. Functional Strength. How do they differ and why is that important?

GK: Absolute Strength is the body's ability to move the greatest amount of weight for one repetition, maximum. For example, chest pressing once and lifting the most amount of weight possible for one time. Functional strength is transferable to everyday activities, like putting a box up on a top shelf. Doing just seated shoulder presses won't do the trick. We need strength throughout our body to get that load up onto that high shelf. We need to workout our shoulders in conjunction with our legs and core since all of those muscles and body parts are engaged in that activity.

SimplyAgeless411: What is your suggested fitness routine for growing younger and stronger physically?

GK: Generally speaking, your fitness routine should consist of the following:

1) Flexibility work through passive, active and dynamic stretching.
2) Resistance training for building strength that has you moving through all planes of motion, while putting an emphasis on stability and core work.
3) Cardiovascular "interval" training that challenges your endurance and works out the heart and lungs.

The goal of a good fitness regimen is one that focuses on strength, muscle building, flexibility, core work, better balance, stability, and mobility. Along with this comes a focus on good posture, a healthy gait, enhanced energy and vitality.

__SimplyAgeless411__: We have heard anti-aging physicians talk about the brain-body connection. They say weak muscles weaken the brain's ability to perform well. Would you explain that?

GK: The greater neuromuscular strength and efficiency you have, the "healthier" you will be. By the way, let me define neuromuscular efficiency a bit better. Think about it as your body's connection to your brain. Your brain sends a signal to make a muscle innervate. If that connection is strong, then your muscle will be able to contract better and do exactly what your brain wants it to do. If that connection is weak, the muscles will not respond as well or as quickly. This is where injury can occur. The more neuromuscular work a person does, the more efficient the brain becomes. That is why many good trainers ask their clients to focus on the muscles they are engaging in any particular exercise: mind over muscle. This actually helps the client to build muscle mass faster with less work, as the brain is engaged in the workout.

__SimplyAgeless411__: How do we reverse sarcopenia and osteoporosis through exercise?

GK: To be specific, resistance exercise plays a huge role in the reversal of sarcopenia and osteoporosis. For those that don't know, sarcopenia is the degenerative loss of muscle mass and strength as we age. Osteoporosis is the loss of bone density over time. Resistance exercise uses the concept of load and gravity to increase strength. When we workout with weights, we are slowly but surely causing micro-tears in our muscles. In essence, we're breaking our muscles down. After we workout, the body begins a complex series of steps to fix the "damage" we've done and to prevent us from doing that to ourselves again. The body will repair tissue damage and help create more tissue so that it can handle the load put upon it.

The same in essence can be said when it comes to our bones. Resistance training has been shown to increase bone density in people over and over again. Gravity plays on the bones of our bodies. As we increase the load on our skeletons, the body needs to adapt to the extra "weight". It then helps create greater bone density to handle the increased load. With proper and consistent weight training, sarcopenia and osteoporosis can be reversed in due time.

SimplyAgeless411: I have been told that weight training, in and of itself, makes the body contract. Doing this repeatedly without other flexibility, core and balance training can cause muscle pain, knots and spasm that can worsen over time. What do you do with your clients to avoid these "weight lifting issues"?

GK: Again, I believe in integrative exercise, which by its nature is expansive. Many of my clients who have never trained this way before report a greater sense of well-being, more relaxed muscles, relief from many of their aches and pains. I incorporate movements that stretch the body while building strength and stamina. I also am a strong believer in "circuit training," which helps elevate the heart rate, helps you burn more calories, and builds endurance. Circuit training is a series of exercises that incorporates weight resistance with cardiovascular training, and keeps the heart rate elevated for as much of the workout session as the client can comfortably tolerate. This type of training seems to yield the best results in terms of better health and a more aesthetically pleasing body.

SimplyAgeless411: Is it okay to be a "weekend warrior"? What are the possible dangers of doing this?

GK: Obviously any exercise is better than none, but the concept of a weekend warrior lends itself to possibly injury. Let me introduce you to the Law of Adaptability. This law basically states that our bodies will adapt to continuous stimuli over a period of time.

As weekend warriors, we spend most of the weekdays sedentary. We sleep. We wake up and sit in our cars on the way to work. We sit all day at work. We sit in our cars to go home. We then sit in front of the TV or computer before going to bed. Our bodies will ADAPT to that lack of activity, and to the positions we continually put them in.

The weekend comes and the "weekend warrior" jumps outside to play tennis, golf, basketball etc, activities they haven't been doing for a long period of time, nor have they been moving at speeds required to be successful at these sports. Because their bodies are used to being more inactive, the possibility of getting hurt is higher. The body isn't as prepared to react quickly. What often happens are torn ligaments, slower motor skills and a greater tendency to fall because your body isn't as stable on its feet because it's gotten comfortable sitting down.

It's ironic that developing nations tend to have less incidences of joint problems and injury than in cultures likes ours, because they have to live and work in a much more active, manual labor environment. There is much less obesity, if any. Their daily routines are working every muscle from head to toe, and their bodies stay younger and healthier. Americans seem to be the most sedentary society as a whole. We drive to work, sit all day, then come home and sit in front of our computers or television sets and consume large, processed meals that are laden with pesticides and preservatives. If we do work out, it is often isolated exercise and then sitting again. The worst offender is the weekend warrior, where the most injuries occur.

SimplyAgeless411: Can aging be reversed in regard to muscle tone, flexibility, and strength?

GK: Most definitely aging can be reversed. The concept of "aging" is couched in cell degradation. "Our bodies break down as we get older" is the common refrain. But really, with proper nutrition and exercise, aging can be stopped in its tracks. I know people that are 50 chronologically but have the heart, lungs and joints of a 30 year old. Like the old saying, "aging and feeling old is a state of mind."

Action Plan
for Diet and Exercise

In Your 20s: This is the time of your life to consciously build a solid foundation for your health, fitness and wellness. Learn about eating natural fresh foods, hormone free proteins, pesticide free fruits and vegetables. Read food labels! Follow the 40/40/20 plan for balanced eating and optimal wellness: 40% carbohydrates, 40% proteins, 20% good fats at each meal. Eat three light meals and two to three snacks per day. Limit soda, alcohol and caffeine intake. Keep fast food and processed foods to an absolute minimum.

Exercise should focus on weight lifting and learn good form now while you are young. Do intense cardio and yoga (or other form of stretching). Since most people who are in their twenties finish their education and enter into the workforce, they need to consciously make exercise a part of their daily routine. This is the time to get into good habits that will serve you well for a lifetime. The goal is to get into the best shape you can. Slim, muscular and full of energy to look and feel great.

At the age of 25, muscle mass loss begins. The average person will lose 1 ½ lbs of muscle mass per year if they don't do consistent weight resistance training. What you do now will affect how you age in later years.

In Your 30s: Resist the temptation to exist on caffeine and sweets. During these busy career building years when most people start their families, you are at risk for putting your health last. This is when you need great nutrition to give you a balanced sense of well-being and extra stamina. Focus on healthy snacks, plenty of water with lemon, and eating every balanced meals every two to three hours. Do not overeat. Learn to be satisfied feeling 80% full. Moderation is the best habit to form in your thirties.

Since time for exercise may be minimal, you should aim for high intensity cardio for 45 minutes, four to six days per week. Spinning, running, and the elliptical are all recommended. Continue with weight resistance training three times per week to avoid muscle mass loss, focusing on your upper body strength. Stretching now is crucial to lower your stress levels. Yoga is highly suggested.

Make good health habits part of your family routine. Jog with your children in their strollers. Hike together. Ride bicycles. Stay active any way you can while you teaching your children the importance of good health. Be a great role model. For those of you that do not have children, continue to make your health a priority. Avoid becoming a weekend warrior.

In Your 40s: Understanding how your individual body type metabolizes food will help you stave off the ravages of aging. DNA testing and/or understanding your blood type are effective ways to identify the right diet for your body type. Modifying your eating habits in this more individualized manner will keep you leaner easier. When eating at restaurants, focus on simply grilled proteins, steamed vegetables, and large salads. Avoid heavy sauces and fancy dressings...opting for fresh olive oil and lemon instead. A glass of red wine is healthy for your heart and stress reduction. Eat plenty of omega 3 oils and aim to make your meals as colorful as possible: a wide variety of fruits and vegetables provide a large spectrum of nutrients.

Weight resistance training is more important now than ever. This will keep your body looking young and your bones strong. Begin learning about integrative exercise that challenges your brain, builds balance and enhances your mobility. A good stretching regimen is crucial for avoiding joint problems later in life. Be aware of your posture and do exercises that build your back muscles and open your chest muscles. Standing up straight will make you look younger and more energized.

In Your 50s and Beyond: Focus on eating regenerative foods. Super greens powders, wheat grass, fresh green juices, anti-oxidant juices, omega 3 and 6 oils, whole grains, lean proteins, and colorful organic fruits and vegetables. Eat foods that make you feel good and look good. This is the time to bring back your glow! Eat to be very healthy, slim and full of vitality. This can be the best time of your life if you are healthy.

Exercise now must focus more on feeling good than looking good. Integrative exercise with proper form is crucial. Getting a personal trainer would be a wise investment. Walking and hiking will give you added endurance and a rosy complexion. Weight training, isometric exercises, core strengthening, flexibility movements, multi-planar movements, and resistance exercise will give you a stronger, toned, and more youthful body. Combination exercises should challenge your brain and mind/body connection. The goal is to be pain-free and independent for the rest of your life.

PART VII

A New Age Is Here...

New Frontiers & Breakthroughs in

AntiAging & Regenerative Medicine

Chapter Twelve

Breakthroughs in Anti-Aging & Regenerative Medicine

Over the past half-century, we've split the atom, we've spliced the gene, we've reached for the stars, and never have we been closer to having them in our grasp. New science and new technological breakthroughs are making the difference between life and death.

Between 2010 and 2025 the race for genetic enhancements will be what the space race was in the 20th Century—genetic therapies and biomedical enhancements will be a multibillion-dollar industry. New techniques will enable doctors to change your DNA to revitalize old or diseased organs, enhance your appearance, increase your athletic ability, and boost your intelligence.

We envision a new world order in medicine, one in which the medical profession creates a new cadre of practitioners out of our medical schools who are preventive integrative health specialists rather than disease specialists.

Adult Stem Cells – Mending Broken Hearts and Much More

From robotic limbs to plastic joints, some doctors describe today's rapid-fire breakthroughs in adult stem cell therapy as nothing short of a miracle. Unlike the more controversial embryonic stem cell therapy, adult stem cells are taken from the patient's own blood and then reintroduced into the patient to treat a number of conditions, including congestive heart failure, peripheral artery disease, coronary artery disease, kidney disease, pulmonary disease, macular degeneration, early dementia. And... this is just the beginning.

Dr. Zannos Grekos, a cardiologist and lead researcher at Regenoctye Therapeutic, spoke at the 16th Annual World Congress on Anti-Aging in Las Vegas, and SimplyAgeless411 was there.

"We've already made significant progress in treating diseases that were thought to be untreatable," Dr. Grekos told the crowd. "The results of our experience with adult stem cell therapy show the potential for use in every aspect of human pathology. This will radically change the way that physicians approach and treat patients in the future." **Regenocyte Therapeutic** (www.Regenocyte.com) was the first clinically treating stem cell

center based in the United States. Its international team of Board
Certified physicians and scientists use adult stem cells taken
directly from the patient's own blood or bone marrow to treat
serious health conditions. Their cutting edge technology, advanced
protocols and cooperation with major medical research centers like
Mayo Clinic, University of Florida and Mayo Clinic have gained
recognition worldwide as leading Regenerative Medicine into the
future.

Immediately following the presentation, more than two dozen
physicians eager to learn more about Dr. Grekos work approached
him in the hallway outside the auditorium. The group was
particularly fascinated with the center's research that proves adult
stem cells already have the ability to engraft themselves into areas
damaged by heart attacks and turn into new heart cells and new
blood vessels.

"Three months after treatment, cardiac nuclear scans of the
areas treated reveal reversal of damage," he explained. "In some
cases, it's virtually impossible to identify the problems that existed
before therapy. We have shown such improvement in some
patients that they were taken off the heart transplant list."

In adult stem cell therapy, a patient's stem cells are extracted
through a simple blood draw at the Regenocyte Clinical Center in
Florida. The sample is sent to a biotechnology laboratory, where

the cells are cultivated and pre-engineered into millions of cardiac regenocytes (living heart repair cells). The patient receives injections of the new cells one week later at one of the clinic's internationally licensed treatment centers. Over the next few months, the cells stimulate tissue re-growth and create greater blood flow to the affected areas. Unlike surgically implanted devices, medications, or organ replacement surgery, using a patient's own stem cells to rebuild damaged heart muscles means there is no possibility of rejection or tumorgenicity (cancer.)

Dr. Grekos and his colleagues in the world medical field are currently employing adult stem cell therapy and coordinating its application for thousands of American patients who have exhausted all other traditional therapy options

Telomeres: The Molecular Timekeepers

Telomeres are the string of pearls at the end of our DNA strain; as we grow older that string grows shorter. But some members of the medical community maintain that telomeres can be regenerated, and strengthened, resulting in substantial increases in vitality and human life expectancy

Living to be 125 may sound like something conjured up in science fiction, but some doctors are saying it's a scientific fact.

And, we're not talking frail, barely-alive 125, but healthy, vibrant centenarians who've achieved the ultimate in being simply ageless. Thanks to recent discoveries about the properties of telomeres and the role they play in aging and how they can be applied toward anti-aging, living well beyond the 100-year mark is within reach.

"For the first time in history, we can now assess the biological age of a human being through telomere testing," says Dr. Mark Houston, a triple board-certified cardiologist, the author of four books and a clinical professor of medicine at Vanderbilt University Medical School. "By making the right lifestyle and nutritional choices based on one's biological age, we can live approximately 125 years." Dr. Houston provided a list of what we can do to maintain a healthy telomere string:

1. Eat a healthy and calorie controlled diet commensurate with your height and weight.
2. Fast 12 hours per day, four days out of the week (example from 6 p.m. until 6 a.m.) Fasting enhances growth hormone and testosterone levels and lowers insulin and cortisol levels.
3. Exercise one hour each day, consisting of 40 minutes of resistance training and 20 minutes of cardio.
4. Get seven to eight hours of sleep each night
5. Take nutritional supplements including Omega 3s, Resveratrol and Green Tea & CoQ10

6. Ideal BMI composition of less than 22% fat for women and less than 16% fat in men

7. Maintain blood pressure of 120/80

Telomeres are confounding the natural laws of aging and the way we heal. Advances in stem cell research are also paving the way for a life expectancy that no one would have believed 20, even 10 years ago. The use of stem cells are not only prolonging life, but in many cases saving it, creating an enhanced quality of living for patient suffering from chronic diseases that they have never known before.

"Telomeres are the body's aging clock," explains Robert Lanza, chief scientific officer of Advanced Cell Technology in Worcester, Massachusetts. Lanza has successfully used stem cells to re-grow the length of the telomere string, which in turn, allows modern medicine to set new precedents in the treatment of illness and aging.

One of the world's top cloning specialists, Lanza experienced early success in his research by copying the genetic material of two rare breeds of oxen from DNA that had been frozen more than 20 years. After cloning herds of cows and comparing their genetic makeup, Lanza studied their telomeres as an entrée into understanding aging in all living things, including humans. What he discovered was that the cows he had cloned had a telomere string that was much longer than their biological parents, meaning their life expectancy was much greater. In short, he had created potentially the world's longest living cows. When applied to humans, Lanza's discoveries could result in men and women reaching ages as high as 180!

"We're really on the beginning of a new medical revolution," Lanza says. "I think with new technologies -- going in and using the stem cells that we were starting to develop - it is possible to prolong human life to several hundred years." Lanza certainly has no plans to clone entire human beings - that's the stuff of science fiction. But his discoveries mean that human cells can be replicated in a lab to repair damaged tissue and provide replacement parts for transplant patients who otherwise could spend years waiting for a donor match.

"We've developed a technique where you can just take one cell, create these embryonic stem cells and not harm the embryo in any way," he explains. "There's a new discovery that was just reported that we can actually take a skin cell, or even a cheek swab, and just turn it into stem cells directly in the laboratory."

Unlike embryonic stem cells, stem cells in adults are predetermined to grow into cells for certain parts of the body. No human embryos are harmed in the course of collecting stem cells.

"The adult body has stem cells in all of your tissues," Lanza continues. "We can get stem cells from fat, we can get them from your brain and we can get them from your skin. Throughout the body right now, there are stem cells that are repairing vessels, they're repairing tissue in your brain. That's how you stay healthy. As you get older and cells die off, you need to replace them with new cells, which is what my research supports is now quite possible." For Lanza, stem cells are a solution to science because they are multipurpose in answering calls from all parts of the body.

"These are the body's master cells," he says. "They're actually immortal. They grow forever. And we can turn them into virtually every cell in your body." Patients suffering from Parkinson's, Alzheimer's Disease, diabetes, atherosclerosis (hardening of the arteries) and strokes could simply exchange their diseased cells for what is essentially brand new, healthy custom-made cells. Lanza says he's even on the verge of research that could eliminate the need for blood donations.

Anthony Attala, director of the Institute for Regenerative Medicine at Wake Forest University, successfully implanted human bladders grown in a lab into seven patients. He used the patients' cells to grow the bladders so there was no risk of rejection. Thirty other patients began clinical trials last year to further study the approach.

"We can actually grow these up by the billions," says Lanza. "So we can create, say for instance, an entire heart or kidney some day, not just bladders. And some day, if you get into an auto accident, we can just take a skin cell and grow you up a new kidney. We're doing this today," he insists. "It's not science fiction."

The science of telomeres has become so mainstream that even Oprah Winfrey declared on her popular talk show that she wants her "telomeres longer." There is a greater understanding now more than ever before that the ability of the cells to divide, to replicate, are what prevents aging. If cells cannot divide, you age. It really is that simple.

Telomerase

Getting that longer telomere string and keeping it healthy is where telomerase plays a substantial role. Already heralded in some medical circles as the "new fountain of youth," telomerase is an enzyme that extends telomeres. The gene that codes for it is part of every cell is the human body, but it can be suppressed or "switched off" in normal cells. In adult stem cells, it is regulated in such a way that it is expressed, but not enough to stop gradual telomere erosion as those cells divide over the course of our lives.

As recently as April of 2010, Telomerase Activation Science Founder Noel Thomas Patton addressed a crowd and extolled the virtues of a remarkable new product that switches that telomerase enzyme "back on," producing dramatic effects on how the body ages.

"Longer telomeres mean a longer life," he said in his presentation. A shorter telomere string can be, to put it bluntly " a kiss of death." Keeping telomeres long is a matter of leading a healthy lifestyle, to be sure, but activating the somewhat dormant telomerase enzyme is key. A molecule identified by Patton's research team called TA-65 effectively does just that. It activates the enzyme that keeps the telomere string long and can be prescribed as a nutraceutical capsule by licensed physicians and rejuvenation specialists.

Telomerase activates certain cells and lengthens telomeres and/or slows their rate of loss. "It allows the cells to live longer in a more youthful state," Patton explained. Users of a prescription-grade telomerase supplement have seen "significant" improvements in immune function, bone density and sexual performance, among other key areas, so much so that many in the rejuvenation field have called TA-65 "the holy grail" of anti-aging.

"For the first time in man's age-old quest, something has the potential to extend maximum human lifespan," Patton reported. There are many that have been taken the TA-65 supplement for as long as three years already, with little no side effects, and numerous benefits, including its ability to fight cancer.

Who should take TA-65? Patton recommends anyone over 40, especially those who have had their telomeres measured and discovered the string is short. For more on this fascinating subject and how telomerase can become part of your anti-aging regimen, see the presentation in its entirey at http://www.tasciences.com/introduction-to-telomere-science/videos.

Human Genomics – You & Your Genome

Your body contains 50 trillion tiny cells, and almost every one of them contains the complete set of instructions for making you. These instructions are encoded in your DNA. DNA is a long, ladder-shaped molecule. Each rung on the ladder is made up of a pair of interlocking units called bases, that are designated by the four letters in the DNA alphabet - A, T, G and C. The long molecules of DNA in your cells are organized into pieces called chromosomes. Humans have 23 pairs of chromosomes.

Chromosomes are further organized into short segments of DNA called genes. If you imagine your DNA as a cookbook, then your genes are the recipes. Written in the DNA alphabet - A, T, C, and G - the recipes tell your cells how to function and what traits to express. For example, if you have curly hair, it is because the genes you inherited from your parents are instructing your hair follicle cells to make curly strands.

Cells use the recipes written in your genes to make proteins - just like you use recipes from a cookbook to make dinner. Proteins do much of the work in your cells and your body as a whole. Some proteins give cells their shape and structure. Others help cells carry out biological processes like digesting food or carrying oxygen in the blood. Using different combinations of the As, Cs, Ts and Gs, DNA creates the different proteins - just as you use different combinations of the same ingredients to make different meals.

To make new cells, an existing cell divides in two. But first it copies its DNA so the new cells will each have a complete set of genetic instructions. Cells sometimes make mistakes during the copying process - kind of like typos. These typos lead to variations in the DNA sequence at particular locations, called single nucleotide polymorphisms, or SNPs (pronounced "snips"). The consequences of "typos" in the SNPs can generate biological variations between people by causing differences in the recipes for proteins that are written in genes. Those differences can in turn influence a variety of traits such as appearance, disease susceptibility or response to drugs.

Learning about your DNA can help you to understand a little better why you are the way you are, and alert you to a predisposition that you may have to a certain type of disease. Scientists can now analyze more than 500,000 SNPs in your genome. Genomics testing can help you interpret your genetic information and understand how your DNA makes you uniquely *you*.

The cost of testing has decreased exponentially over the past few years. At one extreme is Knome, Inc. (www.knome.com), a company which offers precise testing of every one of your genes. Because this service is currently priced at $99,000, almost all of us will need to wait a few years to learn our exact genetic makeup. For most of us, a more affordable entry to the world of genomics is by way of SNP testing.

Disease-based panels of SNPs are available from deCODE Genetics (www.decode.com). Panels offered can measure your relative risk of heart disease, prostate cancer, macular degeneration and others. Very affordable genomics testing is available from 23andme (www.23andme.com). For $399 this company will test for 80 common SNPs using only a scraping taken from the inside of you mouth. Genetic susceptibility to diseases such as age-related macular degeneration, asthma, Alzheimer's disease, atrial fibrillation, cancer (breast, colorectal and prostate), celiac disease, Crohn's disease, diabetes, heart attack, multiple sclerosis, obesity, psoriasis, restless legs, and rheumatoid arthritis are included.

Strategies for Longevity & Optimal Health

With an aging and increasingly unhealthy population, issues of longevity and optimal health are more important than ever. It seems that everyone in our society is searching for ways to live longer, healthier lives. At the same time, we're flooded with information about the most effective path to longevity and optimal health. Countless products promise quick cures, and our news media promote sensationalistic stories about short-lived health trends. But the truth is that there are many clinically proven strategies you can use to drastically extend your lifespan and optimize your well-being. Dr. Terry Grossman, a leading expert on anti-aging and life extension provides his recommendations for ageless living:

1.   **Stay Connected** - In the book, *The Blue Zones: Lessons for living Longer from the People Who've Lived the Longest*, author Dan Buettner reported on his five years of research traveling the globe looking for the places where people lived the longest.

- The island of Sardinia off the coast of Italy - has the most male centenarians in the world.
- Okinawa, Japan - has the longest disability-free life expectancy.

- Loma Linda, California - have life expectancies that average 9-11 years greater than other U.S. residents.
- The Nicoya Peninsula in Costa Rica - where middle-aged people have a 400 percent increased change of living to at least 90 years old.

Buettner identified several things that appeared to be common among people in these areas. The most common denominator was that these people surround themselves with others who share their interests and life's purpose. Social isolation is virtually unknown in any of these regions. This is consistent with medical research that has found that being socially isolated is a health risk. Close interpersonal relationships with a spouse or significant other and individuals who share common interests with you keep you happy and add years to your life.

2. **Add Strength Training to your Fitness Program** - Higher levels of hormones are associated with youthfulness and vitality, and as it is well known that hormone levels decline with age, many people turn to HRT to maintain their levels. There are risks associated with some types of hormonal therapies, but as an alternative you can increase the levels of several hormones associated with youthfulness such as testosterone, DHEA and HGH simply by lifting weights.

In a study reported in the *Journal of Applied Physiology*, Kraemer and colleagues found that 62-year-old men who engage in a 12-week program of weight lifting exercise for 45 minutes twice a week were able to raise their testosterone levels to those of 30-year-old men.

3.   **Get a Spect Scan of Your Brain** - Alzheimer's disease affects approximately 4 million people in the U.S. With the aging of the 76 million members of the baby boomer generation, this number is expected to increase fourfold by 2050. New medications such as Exelon can delay the progression of this disease for many years if it is diagnosed early, however, most people are not diagnosed until it is too late. A special type of brain imaging known as SPECT (single photon emission computed tomography) can help. SPECT imaging can reveal changes in the brain years before the onset of symptoms. This procedure has been recognized by the American College of Radiology and most insurers including Medicare will reimburse for testing.

4.   **Measure Your Vitamin D Level** - We now know that Vitamin D is critical to many functions in the body. It has been found to:

- Decrease fracture risk
- Reduce blood sugar in diabetics
- Help prevent colon cancer (and many other types of cancer)

- Reduce chronic pain
- Increase bone density and help revent osteoporosis
- Lower blood pressure
- Prevent Multiple Sclerosis
- Reduce heart attack

5. **Save Your Stem Cells Now** - Research in biotechnology is currently proceeding rapidly with stem cell therapies occupying a prominent place. Adult stem cell therapies have been used with success in the treatment of such diverse conditions as peripheral vascular disease, congestive heart failure, many types of arthritis, diabetes, wound healing and systemic lupus. Historically, the preferred method for collecting adult stem cells was by way of bone marrow aspiration, however, it is a painful process.

Currently, there are companies that offer stem cell collection and storage where they give their clients an injection of medication that causes significant numbers of stem cells to be released from the bone marrow into the circulating blood stream. Patients then undergo a procedure where their blood travels through a sterile closed system that separates the part of their blood that has the adult stem cells. The stem cells are then separated into multiple vials and placed in cryonics storage so they will be available to you anytime you might need them in the future.

Adult Stem Cell Research Gaining Momentum

Just this summer (2010), the Roman Catholic Church issued a statement supporting the stem cell work of Neostem, even joining forces with the company through its Vatican Pontifical Council for Culture to expand research and raise awareness of adult stem cell therapies (there is no such endorsement for embryonic stem cells by the Church, just to be clear).

Still, this is encouraging, even revolutionary news. Together, NeoStem and the Science Technology and the Ontological Quest unit of the Pontifical foundation will work on a variety of activities with the goal of advancing scientific research on adult stem cells and their application in the field of regenerative medicine. The Vatican was especially interested in Neostem's technology of harvesting self-donated adult stem cells that mimic the properties of embryonic stem cells without the issues of rejection or the controversy stirred up in the media.

The weight of the Vatican's political, financial and promotional backing of such technologies is testimony to the valuable, life-affirming role stem cells can have.

Chapter Thirteen

Rejuvenating Your Brain

If you sometimes feel that your brain is getting a little foggy, or you just aren't as mentally alert as you once were, it could be your brain power is running low. Exercise, diet, supplements all contribute to a healthy body, spirit, and yes, mind. They work hand-in-hand for overall well being. If you have two out of three, you're not winning the fight against aging. Making the most use of our brains has far-reaching impacts on how you age and how long you live.

Do we get more forgetful as we age? Sure, it happens, but as we've revealed earlier in the book, there are supplements out there that can stave off those "senior moments." We're conditioned to believe that we're born with a finite number of brain cells, and as we age, cells die and compromise your thinking and memory. But experts reveal this isn't the case.

Yes, brain cells (called neurons) do in fact die, but the brain has the amazing capacity to create new ones, especially those in charge of learning and memory. Stimulating the brain and keeping it active can work wonders, and it can be done at any age – you can train your brain to function better. One such way of doing so is, believe it or not, through playing games. Studies have shown that older adults demonstrated better motor skills, sharper math skills and a greater cognitive function if they enjoyed some sort of game on a regular basis.

In an article in MORE Magazine, Dr. Deborah E. Barnes, PhD, contends that keeping your brain challenged is the key. "If you're engaging in social activity, such as a game, you're stimulating a lot of different aspects of cognitive function at once," she told MORE. "Although (card game) bridge hasn't been studied, I like it because is has all the components of a major brain booster.

It places you in a social setting and requires you to communicate bids with your partners, employing language skills; to remember which cards have been played, using short-term memory, and to strategize your next move, using judgment and expert knowledge. Chess, Scrabble, and even Concentration require some combination of these skills and reasoning and so can have help stave off mental aging." She recommends that you don't do something that's too easy for you, or the brain will get bored. Tackling a particularly challenging game or puzzle and keeping the brain working has been proven to show improvement in patients with Alzheimer's.

Of course, if gaming isn't your cup of tea, any activity that draws gives the brain a good workout is acceptable. Reading, playing an instrument, attending the theatre, learning a new language, taking some sort of class like pottery or flower arranging, can be good for the brain and soothe the soul. Pick an activity you like. If it becomes tiresome or dull, move on to something else. Stay challenged with these tips:

Walk. Research shows that walking reduces your risk of developing dementia and even Alzheimer's disease, possibly because it reduces your risk for hypertension, diabetes, obesity, and mini strokes, all of which are associated with increased odds of those conditions. Preliminary studies suggest that exercise could also lead to the growth of new neurons and connections.

Get Social. If you are a "shut-in", you'll be more likely to develop dementia, perhaps because you don't get enough of the mental stimulation that comes from conversation and social activities.

Eat Blueberries and Red Grapes. "Anthocyanins, the chemicals that give these fruits their deep hue, are absorbed into the brain's membranes and can improve memory and cognition. Frozen fruit works just as well as fresh. Get the same benefits with: plums (fresh or dried), purple grape juice, blackberries, and red cabbage.

An Apple a Day. Cornell researchers recently found that quercetin, an antioxidant in apples, may protect the brain from the kinds of damage seen in diseases such as Alzheimer's and

Parkinson's. All varieties contain healthy amounts of this and other antioxidants. The peel is where the compound is most concentrated.

Meditate. A calm, focused mind also improves memory and concentration. So much of forgetfulness has to do with multitasking, with your mind scattered in a million directions. Meditation teaches you to be mindful in the present moment, letting go of negative spiraling thoughts.

Do a Crossword Puzzle Every Week. Crosswords require memory of past events and words as well as visual-spatial function. Sudoku requires these functions plus logic. Some researchers believe that consistently playing these games may build up what's known as cognitive reserve.

Work Your Brain. Read a magazine. Reading books, magazines, and newspapers several days a week has been associated with a 35 percent lower risk for dementia in older adults compared with those who read less often, according to a *New England Journal of Medicine* study, though researchers aren't sure if a lack of reading caused the dementia to develop or if early dementia caused subjects to stop reading.

Turn up the Radio. Listening to music triggers the release of the feel-good brain chemical dopamine, which in turn promotes storage of memories. New research shows that we're better able to record memories when we're in a positive frame of mind.

Feed Your Mind. Feed your memory the right foods. Eighty percent of the brain is fat, so you need to provide it with the right fats. The most important one is DHA [docosahexaenoic acid]. People who have the highest levels of DHA have the lowest risk of Alzheimer's disease. You get DHA primarily from eating fish or seaweed. If you're watching your fish intake, any DHA supplement that is made from marine algae is perfectly safe. Also, avoid eating bad fats. Processed hydrogenated fats, like trans fats, which are so common in our diets, make for a brain that works less well."

Jump. Aerobic exercise boosts brainpower, including the ability to pay attention to things focus and regain your memory. New research tells us that as little as four months of exercise could give you 100 to 200 percent improvement in your brain power.

Get Into the Game. If you can't remember where you put your keys or forget who you are calling when dialing a number, you can sharpen those skills with such games as Nintendo's *Brain Age* (www.brainage.com) and the *Smartbrain* CDRom System (www.smartbrain.net), both of which include helpful math games.

PART VIII

Final Thoughts

A New Society & *New Era*

We have all heard it a thousand times, "everything begins in the mind". In the field of rejuvenation, the mind plays an important role in achieving a person's goal of growing younger. It is well documented that the mind has the power to heal the body or weaken it. Many American medical doctors are finally acknowledging the mind-body connection in illness as well as in creating wellness.

Almost every person has been told that they were going to age a certain way. These so-called sage "wisdoms" were passed on from grandmother to mother to child. Men did their share of myth-telling too. Because of this, we can say that from a very young age, we have pre-programmed our minds to help our bodies accelerate aging, disease and decline. In other words, it's what we learned to expect and rightly so for that time in history. No wonder so many people are depressed about aging. They bought into these myths and even now so many people have not updated their data about aging.

So, let us think about aging more logically and with a fresh outlook. If you think about aging logically, it can be an honor, not a horror, to age, especially to age well. When something becomes an honor, we tend to it with care. That's exactly the kind of mindset we need to begin being ageless, vibrant, and healthy.

We need to honor the aging process, understand it and then do what it takes to age well. The result of which is an active, independent and joyous life. Plus you can choose to look great too! No, you probably won't look 29 forever, but you can have good skin tone, white beautiful teeth, strong muscles and bones, good health and a strong mind. You can also enjoy an active sex life as long as you choose to. Yes, you can!

Our thinking about aging is antiquated. It's as if our way of thinking hasn't caught up yet with the technological medical advances that are now available. That's almost the same as thinking that everyone still has to go to the library for information and data, rather than look things up on a computer. Libraries are great, but nothing delivers data faster than a computer. Most people's thoughts about aging aren't in alignment with the new way to age. There's a huge time warp between the recent advances in anti-aging integrative medicine and people's belief systems, knowledge and data.

In many ways, the general population's idea of aging is archaic. Understandably, due to the lack of acceptance of anti-aging medicine by the general medical community, which is slow to embrace new modalities, even at it's own peril. Almost all of us remember when the AIDS virus was discovered. Researchers told medical doctors that they suspected the virus was spread through the blood. But doctors refused to listen. The Red Cross continued to give blood transfusions without checking the blood source to see if it was HIV positive.

Thousands of innocent people contracted HIV because of the refusal to blood test donors or the existing blood bank supply. This is because it takes on average 15 years for the AMA to accept embrace and integrate new treatment modalities or fields of medicine. Fifteen years! Can you imagine waiting 15 years to try a new cell phone or computer program? Can you imagine being told to wait 15 years if your health was severely threatened? We don't always have 15 years.

It is mostly the integrative medical doctors, anti-aging doctors, and gynecologists who have pioneered the new field of regenerative/longevity medicine. Unfortunately, they are still a relatively small group. They endure ridicule from the AMA at large. Anti-aging medicine is aimed at creating enhanced wellness, vitality, and longevity. In other words, it seeks to create homeostasis and keep people living healthy long lives…as drug free as possible.

This is contrary to the AMA's general philosophy of the overuse of "prescription" medications. Natural hormone replacement, supplementation with vitamins and minerals, are a large part of the anti-aging protocol, not pharmaceutical drugs. Regenerative Integrative medicine seeks to rebalance a person's health and vitality, thereby regenerating their cells. Wellness is the primary goal and it is totally achievable, again contrary to popular belief.

We can't help but wonder if we are being kept in the dark about the new technological, medical and cosmetic procedures that rejuvenate the body. Why isn't more being done to educate the public and raise awareness about the world of age management? Age management is not "senior day care centers" or "social security". Age management is the new medical field of anti-aging and rejuvenation. True age management is educating the masses so they can live long, healthy, productive lives with the mindset that good health is natural and right, not illness. Most importantly, it is proactive, not reactive in its fundamental belief system.

The "baby boomers" are the largest segment of our population. They are also the first generation of adults to continually educate themselves well past the "official" school years. Open to new ideas, they seem to be the trailblazers for anti-aging: because of the need and the mindset. Even so, only a small percentage of them truly understand what is available to them in terms of regenerative medicine. Someday, age management and rejuvenation will be commonplace and considered part of standard medical protocol. Now it is a field that is largely misunderstood, feared or laughed at. It's as if we are living in the age of light, shrouded in darkness!

There is no reason for us to age the way we have been aging. Disease, frailty, flabbiness, stooped over posture, instability, pain, loss of sexual vitality, memory loss and more do not need to be our average experience. No wonder most people dread aging. Our fear is so large that we even make fun of birthdays starting age 30 as being "over the hill" or saying that "it's all downhill now".

In the United States, we revere youth and disdain the elderly. We outsource our productive workers as they move into their forties or fifties for younger employees. We make fun of the elderly, push them into old age homes, and ignore them as if "aging" is a disease that may be contagious. It repulses us and makes us uncomfortable. With this mindset of fear, disdain and ignorance, no wonder we age so terribly. We live largely sedentary lives, eat processed over chemicalized fast foods, take too many prescription drugs and treat our elderly very badly.

In other countries, coincidentally, the reverse is true. They eat mostly fresh unadulterated foods, walk most places, use their bodies way more, take much less medications, and have great respect for the elderly. Could there be a connection? Of course there is.

To age differently, we must first embrace aging and then change our paradigm of how we will age. There is a new phenomenon happening. It is a small group of seniors that defying the standard aging process. They are staying physically fit, attractive, well dressed, educated, modern and full of life! They are called "super seniors". People like Dr. Bob Delmontegue, Kelley Nelson, Jack La Lane, and many more.

Centenarians are the first group to defy societal ideas about aging. In Europe, South America, and Asia, the elderly have aged better than in the U.S. for years. This can be attributed to many factors: fresh unadulterated food without chemicals, processing and preservatives, more walking and exercise, respected and admired for their wisdom, seen as a vital part of society, more elegance and style, etc. Rather than being pushed aside, they are exalted for their wisdom and experience.

From a very young age, we have all heard people say, "Well, my body will never be the same after having children" or "After 40, it's all down hill" or even worse, "My mother or father had cancer (or heart disease or arthritis, etc) so therefore, I probably will too". What about those unsettling predictions like, "You can't help but get flabby when you're older" or "When you're older, your body gets stiff and can't move like it used to". Sayings like "I'm too old to learn that or do that!" have become the norm. What's frightening is that people in their early 30s say they feel old!

Myth Busters

Now let's dispel these myths (or old wives' tales as they have been called). Let's look at them one at a time:

1) Flabbiness: is not due to age, but more from a lack of proper exercise, declining testosterone levels, hormone imbalances, low protein diets, poor nutrition, and sedentary lifestyles. All reversible.

2) Stooped over posture: due to lack of muscle tone, core strength, lactic acid buildup, insufficient stretching, laziness and lack of conscious body awareness. Poor ergonomics also play a role in poor posture. Almost completely reversible (or greatly improved) if not caused by an accident or severe illness.

3) Dull complexion: due to lack of essential oils, minerals, and vital nutrients, sluggish elimination, lack of exercise, lack of skin exfoliation and hydration (internally and externally). Can be corrected.

4) Dry, brittle, thinning hair: Usually due to a thyroid imbalance, lack of minerals and vitamins, too much DHT in the bloodstream, not enough essential oils and omega 3/6 fatty acids. Can be greatly improved, sometimes reversed, if treated before the hair follicles die.

5) Large abdominal area/wide waistline: due to poor diet, little to no exercise, over consumption of alcohol, high cortisol levels, hormone imbalances, stress, processed and artificial foods, too much food, sluggish metabolism and lack of sufficient exercise.

6) Genetics: play only a 20-25% role in how we age, contrary to popular belief. The other 70-75% is learned behavior, mindset and lifestyle. We think how we age is genetic, however, much of the time it is more about how we learned to eat, handle stress, think about illness/wellness from our parents. It is a case of "nuture" more than "nature" that determines a person's aging destiny.

7) Tooth decay, tooth loss, and yellowed cracked teeth: This can be a thing of the past. With modern cosmetic dentistry, anyone who has the money can have a beautiful white smile. Proper dental care and nutrition can keep teeth healthy throughout our lifetime, if begun at birth.

8) Hair loss: for males it is most often caused by hormone and nutritional imbalances, low thyroid levels, and too much DHT caused by high testosterone levels. For women, low thyroid levels, low or high estrogen levels, lack of minerals, stress and menopause can cause hair thinning and hair loss. Hair thinning, brittleness, loss of hair elasticity and much hair loss can be reversed if treated before the hair follicles die.

9) Grey hair: now believed to be caused by a lack of certain enzymes in the body such as selenium. Scientists are close to isolating the enzymes that control hair color loss.

10) Diseases of aging: many are due to poor nutrition, lack of weight-bearing exercise, sedentary lifestyles, not enough mental stimulation, stress, mineral and vitamin depletion, lack of hydration, low omega 3 levels, hormone depletion, hormone imbalances, and negative mindset.

Our cells are constantly rejuvenating and growing new cells. In fact, every 21 days we have new cells, every 100 days our cells rejuvenate (either stronger or weaker) with the nourishment they have been receiving, every 7 years we have an entirely new body of cells. Therefore, it is totally logical that if a person started a good exercise program (of weight resistance and cardiovascular strengthening, combined with flexibility training), ate healthier foods, took the right supplements and balanced their hormones, and believed in the power of their body to get better, their body could actually be healthier and better in 100 days. In one year, way better and in 7 years…rejuvenated! Flab could turn to muscle, poor posture could straighten up, dull skin could be revitalized and even hair could be healthier, thicker and shinier.

Every month we meet other people who have also decided to reverse aging. They defy the "norm", the culturally accepted ideas of aging. They look years younger than they are. They have strong healthy bodies and shiny bright eyes. Their skin tone is good and their complexions smooth. They have a nice white smile with beautiful teeth. They have healthy hair. They have a bounce in their step. They look stylish and modern. They are sexually active. They are active and vital members of society. They are happy and have good self-esteem.

As a society, we must change the way we view aging…from seeing it as a shaming disease of decline to a process of renewal, change, hope and wisdom. Only then will we rejoice in each passing year, seeing ourselves as better, more glorious. That does not mean that we will look twenty forever, be it does mean we can be fit, fabulous, healthy, fashionable, and intelligent at any age. As individuals, we must take responsibility for our aging and wellness. By believing that it is normal to be healthy, strong and vibrant we will begin to search out the ways that make it so.

Be careful of what you think and say. Your body is listening. If you don't believe us, believe the Bible, "As you think, so you shall be".

How do you choose to age?

About the Authors

Eve Michaels

As a true testament to what taking control of your life and developing the right anti-aging regimen is all about, Eve Michaels was selected as one of the top 10 finalists for the AARP National "*Model of the Year*" Award.

Eve has more than 30 years experience in the anti-aging, beauty, fashion and image industries and is the creator of the original UK "***Extreme Makeover***". A firm believer that "Knowledge is Power," she has dedicated herself to gathering and sharing information and education with her clients to empower them to make significant changes in their lives.

Passionate about her profession, **Eve** is a highly acclaimed and platform motivational speaker who has addressed thousands on the subjects of anti-aging, beauty and image. Most notable are her image and makeover presentations at multi-speaker seminar events led by the legendary seminar guru, T. Harv Eker, author of *Secrets of the Millionaire Mind*. Engaged in the whole self, Eve also speaks on the importance of adding hormone replenishment, an anti-aging skincare regimen, diet and exercise and anti-aging nutritional supplements to your diet to boost energy and to live a

nutritionally and hormonally balanced life. She is a co-founder
and medical correspondent for *www.SimplyAgeless411.com*, the
national online gateway into the world of anti-aging and cosmetic
rejuvenation and hosts anti-aging bootcamps nationwide.

Eve opened the Nasdaq stock exchange in April 2009 on behalf
of her business, Eve Michaels Enterprises and one of her favorite
charities, The Mannequins, an auxiliary of the Assistance League
of Southern California.

Eve is involved with many charities. The Center Stars, a guild
of The OC Performing Arts Center supports music and theatre
student outreach programs. Her newest endeavor is as a
Motivational Speaker for Working Wardrobes which gives women
and men a second chance to re-enter society with a new corporate
image and skills.

For several years **Eve** worked as an executive cosmetic surgery
consultant for three world class plastic surgeons in Beverly Hills.
As the front line advisor, she provided advice, recommendations
and answers to the myriad of questions consumers had about
surgery and other procedures. In those initial consultations, she
walked clients through every step of the process from beginning to
end. She also hosted informational seminars for those considering
cosmetic surgery and facilitated demonstrations on the latest
techniques and advancements in cosmetic surgery and injectables.

Eve is certified through the Fellowship Program in Functional and Regenerative Medicine through the American Academy of Anti-aging.

On her Simply Ageless partner, Karen Norris:

"Karen tirelessly devotes many hours of time pro-bono every month to helping women and men who are going through the ravages of menopause and andropause. Nothing brings her greater pleasure than seeing people gain the knowledge they need to take responsibility for their health and aging. Karen's tireless research has changed the lives of countless people. Karen's "won't take no for an answer" attitude and determination is a beacon of light in this hurried world."

Karen Norris

Karen Norris - has spent the last ten years researching and consulting with women and men on anti-aging, cosmetic rejuvenation and nutrition. A consummate professional, Karen is *certified* through the "**Fellowship Program**" at the **American Academy of Anti-Aging**, with a focus on anti-aging, functional, aesthetic and regenerative medicine.

Vitamins and nutritional supplements along with bio-identical hormone replacement are at the forefront of her passion and study.

She's spent years researching and interviewing world renowned physicians to identify the most potent and effective hormone replenishment protocol and anti-aging vitamins that are available today. Of special interest are those that can optimize thyroid and hormonal balance for women and men who experience a loss of energy as they approach middle-age.

Through her years as an award winning real estate agent in Beverly Hills, California, **Karen** gained inside knowledge of the "A" list of top physicians and beauty and other medical professionals as well as the coveted anti-aging secrets from her top celebrity clientele. Since then, she has turned her passion for anti-aging into a business consulting firm with her business associate, **Eve Michaels.**

Karen is a co-founder and medical correspondent for www.SimplyAgeless411.com, an online gateway to the world of anti-aging and cosmetic rejuvenation where people have free access to hormone specialists and plastic surgeons around the country and can also interact and buddy-up with each other. They also host anti-aging bootcamps and seminars around the country. As an anti-aging consultant, medical correspondent, speaker, author and, former model, **Karen** knows the challenges and discipline it takes to stay in shape, look good and maintain maximum vitality at every age.

Karen sits on several boards in her community, including the Century City Chamber of Commerce and *The Mannequins* of the Assistance League of Southern California. In 2008 she received the Presidential Award for Volunteerism from *The White House* for her work with the Assistance League, which supports senior citizens and underprivileged children.

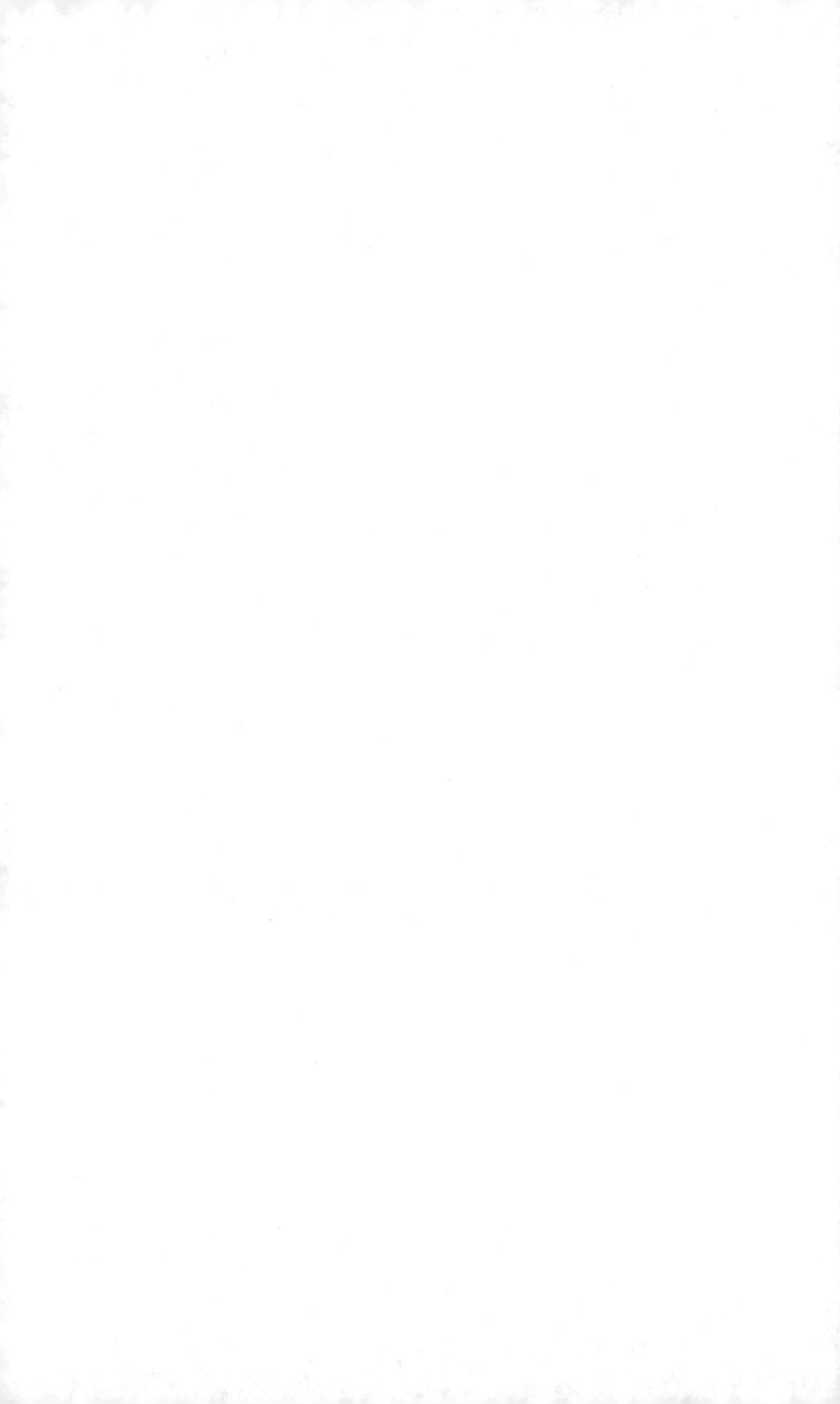

www.ingramcontent.com/pod-product-compliance
Lightning Source LLC
Chambersburg PA
CBHW062124280526
45788CB00001B/47